ALLERGIES AND INFECTIOUS DISEASES

LEISHMANIASIS

SYMPTOMS, TREATMENT AND POTENTIAL COMPLICATIONS

ALLERGIES AND INFECTIOUS DISEASES

Additional books in this series can be found on Nova's website under the Series tab.

Additional e-books in this series can be found on Nova's website under the e-book tab.

PUBLIC HEALTH IN THE 21ST CENTURY

Additional books in this series can be found on Nova's website under the Series tab.

Additional e-books in this series can be found on Nova's website under the e-book tab.

ALLERGIES AND INFECTIOUS DISEASES

LEISHMANIASIS

SYMPTOMS, TREATMENT AND POTENTIAL COMPLICATIONS

CARLOS SEPULVEDA
EDITOR

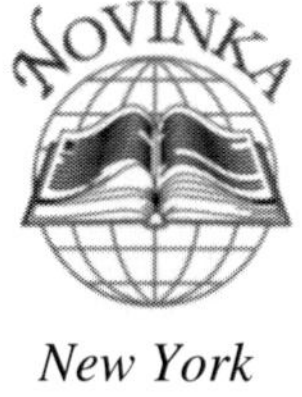

New York

For permission to use material from this book please contact us:
Telephone 631-231-7269; Fax 631-231-8175
Web Site: http://www.novapublishers.com

Library of Congress Cataloging-in-Publication Data

ISBN: 978-1-62417-700-2
Library of Congress Control Number: 2012955269

Published by Nova Science Publishers, Inc. † New York

CONTENTS

PREFACE

The leishmaniases are vector-borne diseases due to infection caused by parasitic protozoans belonging to the Leishmania genus, which find hosts in various wild and domestic animals and can be occasionally transmitted to humans by insect vectors. In this book, the authors discuss the symptoms, treatment and potential complications of leishmaniasis. Topics include immunity against leishmaniasis; the clinical hematology, epidemiology and etiology of leishmaniasis; the role of neutrophils in visceral leishmaniasis; atypical manifestations of canine visceral leishmaniasis; and the parasitological and serological diagnosis of canine visceral leishmaniasis.

Chapter 1 - Leishmaniasis is an anthropozoonotic, vectorially transmitted disease, which is caused by different *Leishmania* species. It is estimated that 350 million people worldwide are at risk of acquiring the disease, which has an annual incidence of 2 million cases. Under the influence of characteristics of the vector, vertebrate host and parasite, leishmaniasis can appear in the cutaneous (localized, disseminated and diffuse), mucocutaneous and visceral forms. In all clinical manifestations, the immune response plays an important role, contributing to the clinical cure or disease progression. Components of innate and acquired immunity act dynamically attempting to control the infection, so the host can achieve clinical cure.

Considering these aspects, this chapter describes the functions of some important elements in innate and acquired responses against *Leishmania* (i. e. chemokines, co stimulatory molecules, receptors, cytokines and cells) in the different clinical forms of leishmaniasis.

Chapter 2 - Leishmaniasis occurs commonly in four continents and is considered to be endemic in 88 countries. Like many neglected diseases, leishmaniasis has a focal distribution and occurs in remote locations. It is a significant public-health problem, endemic in 88 countries, 72 of which are developing countries. In 2007, the Sixtieth World Health Assembly, WHO's decision-making body, adopted Resolution WHA60.13 regarding the control of leishmanaisis: it discusses the impact on disease-control issues, activities in the areas of screening, diagnosis and treatment, and the search for more effective medicines, underlying factors of failure to control disease, including an update of epidemiological information. Recent WHO reports updating epidemiological data indicate that the core problem of leishmanaisis is the access to treatment. Here the authors focus their attention on reviewed epidemiology, clinical presentation, diagnosis and currentlyavailable treatment options.

Chapter 3 - Visceral Leishmaniasis (VL) is endemic in Brazil and has great economic and social impact. Each year, approximately 3,156 cases are recorded, with 10% mortality. The most important reservoir is the dog, which is an excellent model for the study of VL. VL is immune mediated, and most studies are directed toward the understanding of acquired immunity, both humoral and cellular. More recently, the role of innate immunity in VL has been the target of investigations. Neutrophils are the major leucocytic cell effectors of the innate immune response because in the course of VL, neutrophils are rapidly recruited to the site of parasite inoculation, but their role in the modulation of infection is not well defined. Neutrophils secrete lytic enzymes and nitric oxide, which cause the death of many pathogens, thus participating in the elimination of microorganisms by phagocytosis, which is mediated by opsonins, the Toll-like receptor family, and lipopolysaccharides. The activity of neutrophils in Leishmania infection has been studied in murine models of the cutaneous form of the disease and appears to play a protective role by killing the parasites in the acute phase but not in chronic infections. In vitro experiments with human neutrophils infected with *L. donovani* demonstrate that the death of intracellular parasites is carried out by the H_2O_2-peroxidase-halide system. BALB/c mice infected with *L. donovani* and depleted of neutrophils show an increase in the number of parasites in the spleen and bone marrow and a reduction of the formation of granulomas in the liver, with a reduction in nitric oxide synthesis. The immune response against the parasite in the absence of neutrophils is altered with increased IL-10 and IL-4 in the serum and spleen and a decrease in CD4+ and CD8+ T cells producing IFN, suggesting that in the absence of neutrophils, the Th1-type immune response is compromised. Moreover, *Leishmania* may use the neutrophil as a mechanism of escape when phagocytized in non-lytic compartments that present markers of the endoplasmic reticulum and are unable to merge with lysosomal organelles. The lpg1 and lpg2 genes, which encode *Leishmania* phosphoglycans, are clearly involved in the ability of the parasite to remain in these compartments, preventing their degradation and delaying neutrophil apoptosis to increase their life span in the cells. In vitro, co-incubation of polymorphonuclear neutrophils (PMNs) with promastigotes of *L. major* leads to the inhibition of the spontaneous apoptosis of neutrophils, resulting in intracellular survival of the parasite. After infection, PMN eventually undergo apoptosis. Phosphatidyl serine is exposed on the surface of apoptotic PMN, leading to their recognition and phagocytosis by macrophages and thus contributing to the maintenance of infection. The aim of this review is to perform a critical analysis of various factors involved in the participation of neutrophils in VL.

Chapter 4 - Leishmaniasis is an important zoonosis worldwide. The domestic dog is the most important reservoir in urban areas. Dogs with symptomatic visceral leishmaniasis usually present weight loss, anemia, lymphadenopathy, splenomegaly, hepatomegaly, glomerulopathy, cutaneous lesions, and onychogryphosis. However, atypical manifestations of visceral leishmaniasis have been reported, especially in endemic regions. Ocular changes such as blepharitis, keratoconjunctivitis, and anterior uveitis occur very often, but less commonly, cyclitis, chorioretinitis, retinal detachment, keratoconjunctivitis sicca associated with lacrimal gland lesions, cataract, glaucoma, and orbital cellulitis are also observed in some cases. *Leishmania* spp. has been associated with inflammatory mononuclear infiltrate in the hearth causing myocarditis, in ocular-associated smooth and striated muscles, and in skeletal muscles, causing myositis. Affecting the respiratory system, sneezing with epistaxis was reported, as well as interstitial pneumonia. In the gastrointestinal tract, multiple lesions of the tongue and colitis have been reported. Polyarthritis and osteolytic osteomyelitis have been associated with leishmaniasis affecting the locomotor system. A comprehensive study of lesions in the genital system of male dogs demonstrated a very high frequency of lesions particularly in the epididymis, glans penis, and prepuce. Furthermore, dogs shed *Leishmania* spp. in the semen. Studies in bitches, however, demonstrated that vulvar dermatitis was the only important finding in the female genital system. It is known that dogs with leishmaniasis may present neurological signs. Brain inflammatory mononuclear infiltrate has been described associated with high titers of anti-*Leishmania* antibodies in the cerebrospinal fluid. There are also reports of *Leishmania* spp. causing meningitis and choroiditis. Although cutaneous lesions are often present in dogs with visceral leishmaniasis, unusual manifestations include nodular disease, sterile pustular dermatitis, discoloration of the external nares and nodular dermatofibrosis. The protozoan has been observed associated with canine transmissible venereal tumor. Amastigotes have also been found in a large numbers at other tissues in the absence of lesions. This chapter aims to describe unusual clinical signs and lesions of canine visceral leishmaniasis, and alert clinicians about the importance of including leishmaniasis in the differential diagnosis of atypical manifestations, especially in endemic regions for the disease.

Chapter 5 - Canine visceral leishmaniasis (CVL) is important in the transmission cycle of *Leishmania (Leishmania) infantum* as it constitutes the main reservoir of the parasite in the peridomestic cycle. The authors revise the laboratory diagnosis of CVL since control program in some parts of the world including Brazil has in its guideline the culling of infected dogs based on anti-*Leishmania* antibody detection. But the serological techniques have limitation regarding the specificity and sensitivity. The confirmation of infection is performed by parasitological analysis that is considered the gold standard since it presents 100% specificity. Whereas sensitivity, specificity and predictive values of the parasitological methods are critical aspects for the diagnosis of CVL per se and for the dogs as source of parasite for transmission, parameters that may give indication of this potential are important to unveil. Here the authors discuss the serological diagnosis and then the parasitological diagnosis with focus on neutrophilic infiltrate in the tissue related to transmission potential.

In: Leishmaniasis
Editor: Carlos Sepulveda

ISBN: 978-1-62417-700-2

Chapter 1

IMMUNITY AGAINST LEISHMANIASIS

***Marina de Assis Souza*[1],**
***Maria Carolina Accioly Brelaz de Castro*[1],**
***Andresa Pereira de Oliveira*[1],**
***Beatriz Coutinho de Oliveira*[1],**
***Amanda Ferreira de Almeida*[1],**
***Thays Miranda de Almeida*[1]**
***and Valéria Rêgo Alves Pereira*[1•]**

[1]Laboratory of Immunogenetics, Department of Immunology, Aggeu Magalhães Research Center, Oswaldo Cruz Foundation (CPqAM/FIOCRUZ), Recife, PE, Brazil

ABSTRACT

Leishmaniasis is an anthropozoonotic, vectorially transmitted disease, which is caused by different *Leishmania* species. It is estimated that 350 million people worldwide are at risk of acquiring the disease, which has an annual incidence of 2 million cases. Under the influence of characteristics of the vector, vertebrate host and parasite, leishmaniasis can appear in the cutaneous (localized, disseminated and diffuse), mucocutaneous and visceral forms.

[•]Phone: 55 81 2101 2631, Fax: 55 81 2101 2640, E-mail: valeriaph@gmail.com.

In all clinical manifestations, the immune response plays an important role, contributing to the clinical cure or disease progression. Components of innate and acquired immunity act dynamically attempting to control the infection, so the host can achieve clinical cure.

Considering these aspects, this chapter describes the functions of some important elements in innate and acquired responses against *Leishmania* (i. e. chemokines, co stimulatory molecules, receptors, cytokines and cells) in the different clinical forms of leishmaniasis.

Keywords: Leishmaniasis, innate immune response, cellular immune response

1. Introduction

Leishmaniasis is an anthropozoonotic, vectorially transmitted disease, which is caused by different *Leishmania* species. It is estimated that 350 million people worldwide are at risk of acquiring the disease, which has an annual incidence of 2 million cases.

Depending on some features of the parasite, vector and the vertebrate host, including immunological state, the development of the disease can happen under a spectrum of clinical forms [1]. Localized cutaneous leishmaniasis is the most frequent outcome, being characterized by the presence of one or more ulcerated lesions which tend to self-healing.

In rare cases, the lesions can be numerous due to multiple sand-fly bites or parasite dissemination by blood [2]. In diffuse leishmaniasis, there are several popular or nodular lesions throughout the body surface that can persist indefinitely. The mucocutaneous form is the most aggressive, presenting infiltrative lesions, with ulceration and tissue destruction in the nasal cavity, pharynx and larynx [3].

The appearance of different clinical manifestations is influenced by the host immune response. Thus, the presence of immune effector cells such as macrophages, natural killer cels, CD4+ and CD8+ T cells, cytokines, effector molecules and specific antibodies are critical components to the control of leishmaniasis [4,5,6].

Considering these aspects, this chapter describes the functions of some important elements in innate and acquired responses against *Leishmania* in the different clinical forms of leishmaniasis.

2. Innate Immune Response

Innate responses develop after the initial sensing of invading microbes, leading to the production of effector molecules that contribute to contain initial infection and to mount the subsequent adaptive immune response[5,7].There is growing evidence that the innate immune response mechanisms are also important to the antiparasitic response and infection control[4,7]. We will discuss the aspects of the innate immune response in Leishmaniasis with more details below.

2.1. Contributing Cells

Leishmania life cycle inside the host is dependent upon internalization by phagocytic cells either resident or recruited to the wound site [7]. *Leishmania* spp. has been considered an obligate intracellular pathogen of macrophages, but the parasite also has adapted to live within different host cells than those previously described [8,9].

Neutrophils rapidly infiltrate the skin after *Leishmania* spp. infection, in cutaneous and visceral leishmaniasis, and are present in early lesions being the most immediate responders [9,10]. Both host protective and disease promoting roles for neutrophils have been reported. The protective role of neutrophils is associated with rapid recruitment to sites of tissue damage and pathogen entry, and the subsequent clearance of these recruited neutrophils by macrophage/monocyte populations [10,11]. Active neutrophils kills promastigotes via reactive oxygen and reactive nitrogen species as wells as neutrophils extracellular traps [4,9,11]. However neutrophils are short-lived and undergo apoptosis, and when their corpses are phagocytosed by macrophages it allows silent entry of the parasites into macrophages through direct ingestion of the parasite or through ingestion of parasites that hide outside the dead neutrophils [4,9,12]. These apoptotic neutrophils at infection site may also suppress macrophages functions with the release of anti-inflammatory cytokines such as TGF-β and can cause immune mediated tissue pathology [4,8,9,10,12].

Passage through neutrophils is believed to be temporary, a way of camouflage. Parasites usually can establish infections in macrophages, differentiating into amastigotes that replicate inside parasitophorous vacuole [7,11]. However reports showed that in human visceral leishmaniasis neutrophils can harbor parasites during active disease [11].

Leishmania amastigotes, the intracellular form of the parasite, are able to multiply within macrophages, dendritic cells (DC) and neutrophils [13]. However, it is within mononuclear phagocytes that there is the best evidence for replication and long-term survival of *Leishmania* spp [8]. The resolution of infection with *Leishmania* is associated with presentation of *Leishmania* antigens by macrophages and dendritic cells (DCs) and priming of CD4+ and CD8+ T lymphocytes.

Ultimately, induction of nitric oxide synthase (iNOS) and interferon-gamma (IFN-γ) leads to nitric oxide (NO) production, reactive oxygen species (ROS), and parasite killing by macrophages [4]. The central irony of leishmaniasis is that the macrophage is both the principal immune effector cell charged with killing *Leishmania* amastigotes and also the principal site of parasite proliferation and dissemination [4].

A complex network of immune cells within the skin—dendritic cells, macrophages and Langerhans cells—have a prominent role in cutaneous leishmaniasis, as a bridge from innate to adaptive immune responses [12,13,14]. DCs not only play a key role in the development of a protective immune response to *Leishmania*, but also act as a host cell for the parasites [15].

Resident dermal macrophages are also rapidly infected, and they become the dominant infected population after 24 hours allowing differentiation, growth of *Leishmania spp* [8,11]. These antigen presenting cells engage pathogens and then acquire a mature phenotype, increase their expression of co-stimulatory molecules and then travel along lymphatics to the nearest lymph node, where T cell responses are developed to control infection. In general, accumulation of DCs bearing protein antigen in lymph nodes is found to peak around 24h after inoculation [12,13,14].

Together with phagocytes, NK cells represent the first line of defense against pathogens, working by two principal mechanisms: cytolytic destruction of infected cells and secretion of proinflammatory cytokines. NK cells can be identified at the site of infection as early as 24 hours after *Leishmania* infection [14]. In patients, the amount of NK cells and activity has mainly been related with protection against or healing of disease, and reports from patients with active leishmaniasis (cutaneous and visceral) show that they have a reduction in the frequency of peripheral NK cells [11]. The activation of NK cells in visceral and most likely also in cutaneous leishmaniasis results from the intimate interaction of these cells with dendritic cells, which are triggered by *Leishmania* parasites for the production of IL-12 in a TLR 9 dependent fashion [5].

2.2. Chemokines

Chemokines and chemokine receptors have been shown to have different roles in determining the outcome of leishmaniasis. Chemokines are chemotactic cytokines that coordinate recruitment of leukocytes involved in homeostasis as well as in innate and adaptive immune responses [6,14]. Infection with *Leishmania* induces the expression of a number of chemokine genes in the host. This could potentially be beneficial to the parasite through recruitment of host cells it can infect, survive in and proliferate. In addition to mediating cellular recruitment, chemokines can activate various cell populations, participate in cell mediated immunity and possess anti-leishmanial properties, having roles in adaptive immunity, in macrophage activation and parasite killing [6,14].

Chemokines produced at the site of an infection are critical in determining the composition of infiltrating cells and defining the eventual outcome of the disease [14]. Patients with visceral leishmaniasis show elevated concentrations of CXCL9 and CXCL10 in their serum during active infection and it has been suggested that these chemokines along with IFN-γ play an important immunopathogenic role in the disease [6]. In localized cutaneous leishmaniasis (LCL) a Th1 chemokine profile is observed in the lesions, consisting of CCL2 (monocyte chemotactic protein-1), CXCL9 and CXCL10- associated with a concentrated dermal infiltrate comprising of macrophages and large numbers of CD4 positive cells. In contrast, the chemokine profile of lesions of chronic diffuse cutaneous leishmaniasis (DCL) is Th2 associated, dominated by the expression of CCL3 (macrophage inflammatory protein 1-α), and the dermal infiltrate is more diffuse with fewer CD4 positive cells [9,16].

2.3. Effector Molecules

The key antileishmanial effector molecules in experimental cutaneous and visceral leishmaniasis are reactive nitrogen intermediates (NO and NO-derived metabolites) and reactive oxygen intermediates ($O2^-$ and subsequent metabolites) [5]. While the production of NO is required for the leishmanicidal activity against *L.major* and *L. braziliensis* in the skin of infected mice, it is dispensable in the spleen and mildly important in the lymph node [7].

The entry of *Leishmania* parasite into host macrophages results in the onset of respiratory burst, characterized by the increased production of reactive oxygen species (ROS), like superoxide (O2 -) and hydrogen peroxide

(H2O2), which is required for the killing of the parasites. These O2 - are generated by activities of a multi component enzyme complex i.e., nicotinamide adenine dinucleotide phosphate (NADPH)/NADH oxidase. Moreover, in later stages of infection, reactive nitrogen intermediates (RNI) like nitric oxide groups (NOg) are also produced by the activity of inducible nitric oxide (iNOS), which further contribute to innate immunity and parasitic elimination. However, in leishmanial infections, the microbicidal activities of macrophage are severely hampered, leading to the survival and proliferation of parasites inside the macrophages [19].

2.4. Toll-Like Receptors (TLRs)

The TLR family is highly relevant to immunity against *Leishmania* and other parasites, as they recognize pathogen-associated molecules and participate in innate responses to infections [4,7,19,22]. TLR activation induces innate responses in multiple ways, leading to the production of effector molecules such as nitric oxide, inflammatory cytokines, chemokines, and other anti-microbial products that can directly destroy the pathogens. TLRs are known to participate in the control of *Leishmania* infection by inducing Th1 responses. A few *Leishmania*-derived molecules have been reported to activate TLRs, and the majority of the studies to date focused on the activation of TLR2, TLR4, and TLR9 [7,13,19,22].

Evidences indicate that TLR4 contributes most significantly to control the growth of *Leishmania* spp. in both phases of the immune response. The TLR4 has been found to be a strong regulator of inducible nitric oxide synthase (iNOS, a marker of innate immunity) leading to the death of parasites. In addition to TLR4, TLR2 and 9 have been detected in the skin of patients with cutaneous leishmaniasis [22].

Lipophosphoglycans (LPG) on the *Leishmania* cell surface have been implicated as agonists of TLR 2, 3, 6 and have also been associated with NK cell activation in *L. major* infection [4]. Purified *L. major* lipophosphoglycan induced the upregulation and stimulation of TLR2 on human NK cells, with additional enhancement of TNF-α and IFN-γ. LPGs of *L. major*, *L. mexicana*, *L.aethiopica*, and *L. tropica* were defined as TLR2 ligands in studies using murine macrophages, although the stimulation with *L. tropica* LPG was only marginal. More recently, it was shown that LPG stimulates cytokine production by human peripheral blood mononuclear cells via TLR2 as well.

Those findings assign a protective role for TLR2 which seems required to mount an effective Th1 response [7].

2.5. Complement System

The complement system is a complex set of serum proteins that forms a controlled sequence for the generation of activated molecules. The role of the activated molecules is to increase inflammatory reactions mediated by antibodies.

In addition, generation of the membrane attack complex C5b–C9 leads to the lysis of "unwanted" cells. The complement receptor system is directed against mediators generated by the host right after parasite contact. In *Leishmania* infections the parasites interact with serum and activate complement in both the classical and the alternative pathways. Opsonization of *Leishmania* promastigotes with complement is fast, with lysis by the membrane attack complex beginning seconds after serum contact, resulting in the elimination of more than 90% of the inoculated parasites within a few minutes [13].

2.6. Modulation of Infection in Innate Immune Response

Leishmania parasites are capable of using different components of the host defense innate mechanisms to avoid their elimination from the host before an infection is established. Some of the parasites surface molecules are capable of activating the complement system, resulting in the binding of C3bi and C3b to the surface of the parasite. *Leishmania* parasites smartly use this opsonization to escape from the hostile environment by promoting phagocytosis via complement receptors in cells such as in macrophages, neutrophils and erythrocytes [9,11,13].

They can also entry macrophages using the engagement of non-triggering receptors such the phosphatidyl serine (PS) receptor. *Leishmania* can also evade effector mechanisms of the immune system by direct inhibiting macrophage function through interference with NFB transcription and IL-12 production, disturbing macrophage phagosomal maturation and killing functions. They can additionally down regulate MHC class II expression; promote the production of regulatory cytokines like IL-10 and TGFβ and can inhibit dendritic cell maturation and chemotaxis [4,11,15].

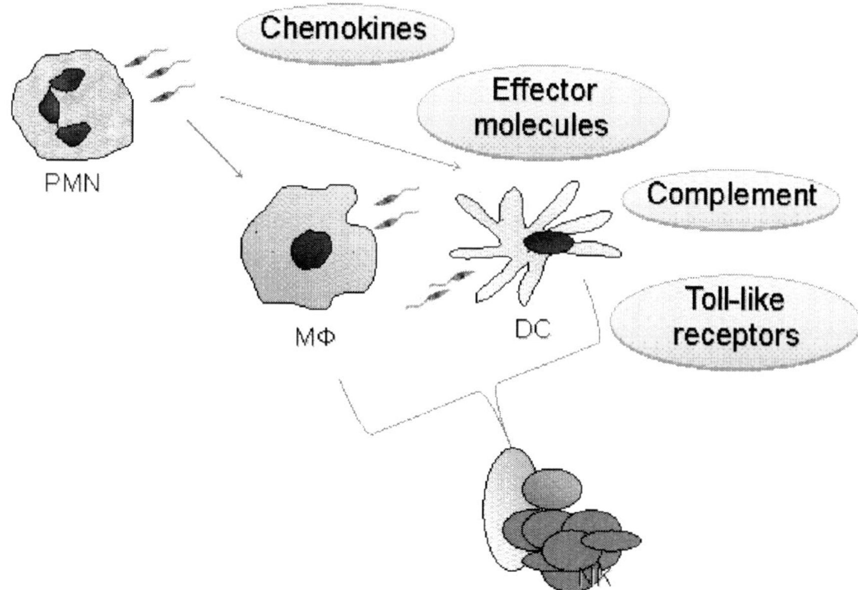

Figure 1. The main components of the innate immune response against Leishmaniasis include some important cells and chemical mediators. Neutrophils are the most immediate responders, which rapidly infiltrate skin after parasite infection. However, it is within mononuclear phagocytes that there is the best evidence for replication and long-term survival of *Leishmania* spp.. Ironically, the macrophage is both the principal immune effector cell charged with killing amastigotes and also the main site of parasite proliferation and dissemination. Within the skin, DCs not only play a key role in the development of a protective immune response to *Leishmania*, but also act as a host cell for the parasites. Together with phagocytes, NK cells represent the first line of defense against pathogens, making cytolytic destruction of infected cells and secreting inflammatory cytokines. The composition of inflitrating cells and the definition of the eventual outcome of the disease are critically determined by chemokines produced at the site of infection. Also, depending on the site of infection, antileishmanial effector molecules play an important role in innate immunity. Composed by a complex set of serum proteins, the complement system is activated in both the classical and alternative ways in leishmaniasis. However, *Leishmania* parasites are capable of using different components of innate defense to avoid their elimination from the host before an infection is established.

3. Acquired Immune Response

In human and experimental leishmaniasis, immunity is predominantly mediated by T lymphocytes. T cells play a major role in generating specific and memory T-cells responses to intracellular parasitic infection and these have been extensively characterized in *Leishmania* infection [25]. In addition, T lymphocytes play critical role in shaping the host immune response by secreting cytokines, which may act both synergistically and antagonistically through complex signaling pathways to direct both protective and non-protective immunities against intracellular parasites [24].

Although the immune response induced by infection with *Leishmania* has been the subject of many investigations, the mechanisms that underlie host resistance and pathogenesis in leishmaniasis are not entirely understood. During the late 80s and early 90s, the discovery of two distinct subpopulations of CD4+ T helper cells based on their cytokine production, Th1 and Th2 [26], finally explained resistance and susceptibility to *L. major* in the murine model [27].

Early studies using mouse models of experimental cutaneous leishmaniasis (CL) have revealed a clear dichotomy between Th1-associated cytokines mediating protection and Th2-associated cytokines mediating susceptibility [23,24,28,31]. Failure to mount an efficient anti-L*eishmania* Th1 response was shown to cause progressive disease and absence of lesion resolution [29,31]. In resistant C57BL/6 mice, resolution of the disease is mediated as a consequence of IFN-γ release by Th1 cells and upregulation of NO in macrophages the harbor parasites [30,31]. Conversely, persistence of lesions in BALB/c mice is due to Th2 –type $CD4^+$ T cell differentiation and production of IL-4, which suppresses macrophage activation, resulting in parasite survival [29,31]. On the other hand, during VL, Th2 response and cytokines such as IL-4 and IL-13 seem to be necessary for immunity and efficient response to antileishmanial chemotherapy [31,32].

In the murine model of *L. major* infection, the predominant $CD4^+$ T cell subpopulation resulting from infection greatly influences the outcome of disease [34,35,36]. Interleukin-12 (IL-12) produced by macrophages and dendritics cells and interferon-gamma (IFN–γ) produced by natural killer cells (NK), and previously activated T cells, promote the development of Th1 cells, whereas IL-4 induces the development of Th2 cells. The Th1 subpopulation, important for induction of leishmaniasis resistance, produce IFN-γ and tumor necrosis factor – alpha (TNF-α) which play an important role in cellular immune responses against intracellular pathogens by activating macrophages for intracellular killing of pathogens[36,37]. On the other hand, Th2 cells produce IL-4, IL-5, IL-10, IL-13 and TGF-β, and are associated with leishmaniasis susceptibility in *L. major* infection murine models [36,38,39,40].

Most data point to the fact that same or similar Th1 dependent mechanisms are involved in control of human disease. Self-healing forms of leishmaniasis and cure of VL is typically accompanied by parasites specific proliferation and IFN-γ production. Human macrophages are activated to kill intracellular parasites by IFN-γ and exogenous IFN-γ can promote cure of human CL [41,45]. Though Th2 responses can act in favor of the parasite, polarized Th2 response has never been able to explain non-curative or visceralizing human disease. Th2 independent disease progression is also supported by studies on non-healing disease in Th1 phenotypic B6 mice [42,45]. In this context it can also be noted that in patients with VL the effect of IFN-γ administration was limited [43,45] and in human LC, IFN-γ production by CD4+ cells, alone, in response to *Leishmania* antigens is not predictive of protection or disease development [44,45]. This indicates that other mechanisms acting in synergy with IFN-γ or counteracting the effects of IFN-γ as important. Thus, the Th1/Th2 dichotomy as an indicator of resistance and susceptibility might be a generalization and is far more complex than what we currently know and understand [31,45].

Of particular interest in this context is the differentiation of Naïve $CD4^+$ Th cells into various effector lineages orchestrating different immune responses. Naïve $CD4^+$ Th cells can differentiate into IFN-γ producing Th1 cells; into Th2 cell secreting IL-4, IL-5, IL-13, and IL-10; or into the recently described Th17 cells. In addition, Naïve $CD4^+$ Th cells can differentiate into IL-10-secreting regulatory T cells like regulatory type 1 T cells, IL-10, and TGF-β producing Th3 cells or into Foxp3-expressing regulatory T cells [46]. Some cytokines are described in the following section.

3.1. Th1 and Th2 Cytokines

To control leishmaniasis infections, activation of macrophages dependent of CD4+ T cell, IFN-γ and tumor necrosis factor (TNF) are usually required. These effector molecules and cells are typically present in a cell mediated immune response. This leads to a (post)transcriptional upregulation of antimicrobial effector mechanisms, including the acidification of the phagolysosomes and the expression of inducible nitric oxide synthase [18,24].

TNF-α is a key cytokine mediating T cell-mediated inflammation. It is involved in leukocyte recruitment by increasing expression of adhesion molecules on vascular endothelium and increasing angiogenesis. Although TNF-α promotes increased macrophage activation, and contributes to control of *Leishmania* parasites, deleterious consequences of excessive TNF-α production have been reported. The high levels of TNF-α and IFN-γ secreted by mononuclear cells from these patients is positively correlated with lesion size and the use of drugs that down modulate production of TNF-α in combination with antimony increases the rate of healing and allows the cure of refractory cases of mucosal and cutaneous disease [15].

The main biological role of IFN-γ is to activate macrophages, inducing iNOS expression and NO production. This contributes to increase the microbicidal activity of these cells and therefore helps in the elimination of parasites and in the resolution of *Leishmania* infection [5,24]. IFN-γ biological effects can be associated with the activation of STAT1 transcription factors. STAT1/IFN-*γ* signaling pathway stimulates the expression T-bet, a transcription factor associated with the Th1 profile. STAT1 and T-bet are considered crucial to host protection against *Leishmania* infection in mice, since they are necessary to mount an efficient Th1 immune response [24].

Type I interferons *α* and *β* (IFN-α/β) are proinflammatory cytokines that are able to activate and phosphorylate STAT1 and STAT2. Their functions in innate and acquired immunity to bacterial and parasitic infections are shown in some studies. IFN-*α/β* can act as early regulators of the innate response to infection and are essential for initiating the expression of nitric oxide synthase type 2 (NOS2) and the production of NO. IFN*α/β* play a critical role in the innate immune response to CL infection by mediating events involved in parasite repression, IFN-*γ* expression, and cytotoxic NK cells activity- all through NOS2. IFN- *α/β* rather than IFN-γ was shown to account for the initial induction of iNOS in the skin and lymph node at day 1 of infection with *L. major*. The task of STAT2 in VL is essentially unknown [5,24].

Known as a proinflammatory cytokine, IL-12 is a heterodimer composed of two subunits, p35 and p40 and is produced primarily by macrophages and dendritic cells (DCs) in response to microbial pathogens. IL-12 functions as the main physiological inducer of gamma interferon (IFN- γ) by activated T cells and promotes Th1-type CD4+ T cell differentiation, and therefore is a key cytokine for the generation of protective immunity in response to *Leishmania* infection. The specific cellular effects of IL-12 are due to the activation of Janus kinase (JAK)-STAT pathways, primarily to the activation of the specific transcription factor, STAT4. In activated T cells and NK cells, STAT4 functions to induce IFN-*γ* production in response to IL-12 signaling [5,24].

IL-10, an anti-inflammatory cytokine, is produced by a variety of cells, such as T cells, monocytes, macrophages, DCs, and B cells. Many other cells can produce IL-10, but its main role seems to be on macrophages and DCs, having a part as an anti-immune and anti-inflammatory cytokine. IL-10 inhibits the production of the proinflammatory cytokines IL-1, IL-6, IL-12, and tumor necrosis factor (TNF), preventing the development of a Th1 profile associated with a protective immunity during *Leishmania* infection. IL-10 also promotes the development of a humoral immune response, with the production of antibodies, which aids parasite entry into host cells. Studies demonstrated that IL-10 is a master cytokine in cutaneous and visceral leishmaniasis that is critical for the initial survival and long-term persistence of *Leishmania* parasites in both human and experimental models. Because IL-10 can act as an inhibitor of IFN-γ induced NO synthesis, it is likely that the antagonistic effects of IL-10 are related to its ability to suppress NO production, a critical component for parasite elimination [18,24].

IL-4 is an important cytokine that has been shown to deactivate macrophages and to regulate the induction of Type-2 [20,21]. Furthermore, IL-4 inhibits the responsiveness of CD4+ T cells to IL-12, due to its down regulatory effects on the expression of the IL-12 receptor b2-subunit and also inhibits the deviation of CD4+ T cells towards Th1 cells by modulation of the regulatory function of the transcription factor T-bet [20,21]. Moreover, macrophage activation by IL-4 induces a pathway of arginine metabolism toward arginase with production of polyamines that enhance *Leishmania* growth [21]. Since IL-4 has been shown to suppress macrophages and Th1 cells and enhances *Leishmania* growth, it is conceivable that the host ability in production of this cytokine may determine the susceptibility to CL. This hypothesis is supported by recent report on the association of IL-4 gene polymorphisms with susceptibility to visceral leishmaniasis [21].

3.2. Regulatory T Cells

To achieve cure in Leishmaniasis, the infected host must develop an immune response capable of eliminating the parasite, but harmless to itself. This balance is given by regulatory T cells, which exhibit two well-defined subpopulations: naturally occurring CD4+CD25+ Tregs, which originate in the thymus during ontogeny, and inducible Tregs, which develop in the periphery from conventional CD4+ T cells [46]. The first subpopulation of Tregs was initially described as a population of CD4+ T cells that prevent the expansion of self-reactive lymphocytes and, therefore, autoimmune disease in mice [47]. This population can be defined by their constitutive expression of the IL-2 receptor α chain (CD25), the cytotoxic T lymphocyte antigen (CTLA4), the TNF receptor family member GITR (glucocorticoid-induced TNF-receptor-related protein), and the a chain of the αεβ7 integrin (CD103) [48]. However, expression of these molecules is not specific to Tregs. In contrast, the forkhead/winged helix transcription factor Foxp3 is thought to program the development and function of Tregs and is specifically expressed in natural Tregs in mice, as well as in $CD25^-$ T cells with regulatory activity [49,50,51].

Cells with regulatory functions have been frequently described in *Leishmania* infections, and the existence of concomitant immunity is discussed [52,53,54]. This phenomenon consists in the long-term persistence of pathogens in a host that is also able to maintain strong resistance to reinfection. In the murine model of infection with *L. major*, $CD4^+CD25^+$ T cells accumulate in the dermis, where they suppress – by both interleukin-10-dependent and interleukin-10-independent mechanisms – the ability of $CD4^+CD25^-$ effector T cells to eliminate the parasite from the site. The sterilizing immunity achieved in mice with impaired IL-10 activity is followed by the loss of immunity to reinfection, indicating that the equilibrium established between effector and regulatory T cells in sites of chronic infection might reflect both parasite and host survival strategies [53].

Regarding the experimental infection with *Leishmania (Viannia) braziliensis*, a Treg activity has also been related. $CD4^+CD25^+$ cells expressing GITR, CD103 and Foxp3 were detected throughout the duration of clinical disease both at the ear and in draining lymph nodes of infected mice. In both sites, they were capable of suppress $CD4^+CD25^-$ proliferation. Interestingly, in the outcome of a reinfection, parasites were mainly detected in the LN draining the primary infection site where a high frequency of $CD4^+IFN\text{-}\gamma^+$ T cells was also present. Thus, in this model, Tregs are present in healed mice but this population does not compromise an effective immune response upon reinfection with *L. braziliensis* [54].

Suppression of T cell response is thought to be involved in the pathogenesis of human leishmaniasis. In patients with CL caused by *L. braziliensis*, a frequency of CD4+CD25+ cells was observed in the skin lesions, along with expression of CTLA-4 and GITR markers and secretion of IL-10 and TGF-β. Moreover, CD4+CD25+ T cells in peripheral blood (PB) from the same patients exhibited higher levels of CTLA-4 than healthy individuals[55]. Because CTLA-4 is highly expressed on Treg cells [56,57], and because it is supposed that this molecule plays an important role in their suppressor function[57], it is possible that the suppressor activity of CD4+CD25+ T cells was increased in the patients with CL.

A similar immune regulation in human visceral leishmaniasis is observed. The presence of CD4+CD25+ in the bone marrow, one of the disease sites, and the production of IL- 10 by these lymphocytes may inhibit T cell activation in IL-10 dependent manner [58]. In contrast, CD4+CD25+ lymphocytes did not accumulate in and were not a major source of IL-10 in the spleen, and their removal did not rescue antigen-specific interferon-γ responses. Thus, in different sites the regulation of immune response may be performed by different T cell subpopulations, once IL-10 is secreted in the spleen by CD25-Foxp3- T cells [59].

It is also interesting to investigate whether there is an influence of mechanisms of immune regulation on the response to chemotherapy. The analysis of the frequency of CD25+ cells in PB from patients with active and cured CL showed a higher presence of cells expressing this marker after treatment. Thus, CD25+ T cell expansion, presented by patients, may be due the role of these cells in the modulation of an exacerbated response by effector T cells, and maintenance of a small number of parasites in the localized lesion as an antigenic stimulus to prevent reinfection [60]. Among all the data obtained so far, immune regulation seems to happen as a way to maintain a homeostatic environment to allow the achievement of clinical cure by the host and the parasite persistence. Nevertheless, conclusive role of Treg cells in suppression of immunity in patients and its consequences is yet to be well defined.

3.3. Th17 Responses in Leishmania Infections

Similar to the Th1 and Th2 subsets, the Th17 subset is orchestrated by specific cytokines and transcription factors [61]. The Th17 response has been studied since 1995, when it was found that T helper cells can produce IL-17 under stimulation with specific antigens [62]. Nowadays, it is known that the production of Th17 specific cytokines is present in allergy and inflammatory diseases [63,64]. However, these inflammatory mediators can orchestrate protective responses to several agents, as it is shown in *M. tuberculosis* and *T. cruzi* infections[65,66].

The Th17 response is activated by a combination of the cytokines IL-6 and TGF-β, and the transcription factors RORγt, RORα and Stat3 are essential for Th17 commitment [60,67]. IL-6 plays an important role in the differentiation of the Th17 subset, since TGF- β can also induce Foxp3, a transcription factor required for the generation of regulatory T (Treg) cells, and the presence of IL-6 suppresses the induction of Foxp3 [67].

Th17 cells produce cytokines such as IL-17A, IL-17F, IL-22, IL-21 and IL-23, which promote Th17 responses functionality. The cytokine IL-27, on the other hand, is the main negative regulator of the Th17 response, despite its structure's similarity to IL-6 [60]. Research over the role of these cytokines in many infections is under constant development. The research of the influence of Th17 cells in leishmaniasis is primordial to understand the mechanisms related to protective or damaging immune responses in this disease. In the next section, some features of these cytokines are described.

3.3.1. IL-17

The IL-17 cytokines include a family of six members (IL-17A-F), of which at least two of them exhibit potent proinflammatory properties: IL-17A (also known as CTLA-8) and IL17-F, which seem to have similar functions. IL-17B and IL-17C are members of the family whose cellular sources are unknown at this point, and whose biology seems unrelated to IL-17A. IL-17D and IL-17E (alternative names: IL-27 and IL-25), in turn, are the two members of the IL-17 family with lowest homology to IL-17A. None of the last is produced by Th17 cells, and they exert a negative control on the Th17 subset development[60]. In this chapter, we will refer to IL-17A as IL-17.

By signaling through the receptor IL-17RA, IL-17 can induce the production of different kinds of proteins, many of them related to inflammation, including chemokines (CXCL-1, CXCL-2, CXCL-8-10, CCL-2, CCL-20), cytokines (IL-6, TNFα, G-CSF, GM-CSF), proteins of the acute phase response, tissue remodeling factors (MMP1, MMP3, MMP9, MMP13, TIMP2), and anti-microbial products (β-defensins, mucins, calgranulins) [60]. The role of IL-17 in immune responses is being widely studied. It is known that IL-17 is a potent activator of neutrophils. Increased levels of this cytokine are responsible for neutrophil immigration, most likely via CXCL2, whereas IFN-γ is responsible for activating macrophages to kill intracellular pathogens [68]. IL-17 seems to have a role in the protective immunity against many bacterial and fungi infections, as in the case of *Klebsiella pneumoniae*, *Mycobacterium tuberculosis*, *Candida albicans* and *Aspergillus fumigate* infections [69,70]. IL-17 could also be defensive against some parasites, as in the infection with the protozoan *Toxoplasma gondii* [71]. Also, IL-17 production appears to be downstream of IL-1αβ in several pathological conditions. DC derived IL-1 is important for efficient Th1 induction in leishmaniasis [68].

Whilst in some models IL-17 and IL-23 seem to have a protective role on the outcome of the infection, as in the case of extracellular pathogens (e.g., *Klebsiella pneumonia* bacteria, *Toxoplasma gondii* parasites and *Cryptococcus neoformans* fungi) [72], in *Schistosoma mansoni* infections, increased levels of IL-23 and IL-17 are associated with disease exacerbation [73].

As to leishmaniasis, Kostka et al (2009) reported that BALB/c mice produced increased levels of IL-17 after infection with *L. major* and that IL-17-deficient (IL-17$^{-/-}$) BALB/c mice exhibited dramatically attenuated disease despite typical Th2 development. They also demonstrate that elevated levels of IL-17A in BALB/c mice were associated with increased production of IL-23, but not IL-6 and TGF-β1, by infected DC.

In humans, studies have shown that IL-17 is present at the initial phase of the immune response in the cutaneous forms of leishmaniasis [68,74,75], leading to the conclusion that this cytokine could be injurious for the disease resolution. On the other hand, Novoa et al (2011) observed an increase in IL-17 levels in individuals with subclinical ACL, in comparison to patients with active lesions, concluding that this cytokine presents a protective part in the immune response. Pitta et al (2009) have also shown that *L. donovani*, a visceral leishmaniasis agent, strongly induces IL-17 and IL-22 production in PBMCs of healthy individuals, suggesting that these cytokines can present a protective role in *Leishmania* infections.

3.3.2. IL-21

Although IL-21 does not look like an essential factor for Th17 lineage commitment, it is able to induce IL-17 expression in collaboration with TGF-β even in the absence of IL-6. Furthermore, generation of Th17 cells is attenuated by blocking IL-21, and loss of its expression, or its receptor, results in defective Th17 differentiation. Similar to IL-6, IL-21 inhibits Foxp3 expression induced by TGF-β. IL-21 is produced by Th17 cells under IL-6 induction and autocrinally induces its own synthesis and the expression of IL-23R to allow IL-23 responsiveness [68].

Furthermore, IL-21 has been recently proven to induce IL-10 production under stimulation with *L. donovani* antigens. It is also known to critically regulate Ig production, and could be a contributing factor to the high titers of anti-leishmanial Abs in VL patients [76].

3.3.3. IL-22

IL-22 is also produced by Th17 cells, and to a lesser extent by Th1 and NK cells, and is involved in immunity at the epithelium and mucosal surfaces

[77,78]. The functional IL-22 receptor is expressed on hepatocytes, keratinocytes, and fibroblasts. IL-22 increases the production of proinflammatory molecules, such as the S-100A proteins and CXCL5. IL-17 and IL-22 synergistically increase the production of antimicrobial peptides, such as β-defensins, by epithelial cells [68,78].

Both IL-17 and IL-22 have been shown to increase protection against certain bacterial and fungal pathogens in experimental models [78]. As to protozoans, Pitta et al (2009) stated that IL-17 and IL-22 are the cytokines most strongly associated with protection in the visceral forms of leishmaniasis. These cytokines may contribute to protective immunity to *L. donovani* in several ways. Studies using animal models suggest that neutrophils could be involved in controlling the *Leishmania* infection through the generation of skin and liver granulomas that form around *Leishmania* at early stages of infection. Furthermore, IL-22 is involved in epithelial repair and liver protection in chronic infections. Both the increases in epithelial protective barrier function and the recruitment of inflammatory cells, including neutrophils, to the skin and liver, could contribute to protection against *L. donovani* [78].

3.3.4. IL-23

The function of IL-23 in promoting Th17 cell expansion or survival has been proposed. A recent report suggests that IL-23 maintains the Th17 phenotype without affecting proliferation or survival. On the other hand, IL-23 has been demonstrated to maintain the pathogenic Th17 functions compared with culture under TGF-β and IL-6, depending on IL-10 production by Th17 cells [60].

Recent studies have also implicated IL-23 and IL-17 in immunity against extracellular pathogens, as bacteria (*Klebsiella pneumoniae*), *Toxoplasma gondii* parasites and fungi (*Cryptococcus neoformans*). In *Schistosoma mansoni* infections, increased levels of IL-23 and IL-17 are associated with disease exacerbation[72]. Kosksta et al (2009) suggests that DC-derived IL-23, in addition to IL-1β and IL-12p80, can contribute to disease susceptibility in BALB/c mice infected with *Leishmania* parasites.

3.3.5. IL-27

IL-27 is one of the main negative regulators of Th17 development. This cytokine is structurally related to IL-6, but has many different actions. Research studies show a damaging role of IL-27 on IL-17 producer cells. These studies conclude that the absence of IL-27 signaling exacerbates chronic inflammation in correlation with increased number of Th17 cells. Moreover,

IL-27 is able to promote IL-10 production, another negative player in the network of Th17 activity regulation [60]. Novoa (2009) reported a higher expression of mRNA for IL-27 *ex vivo* or in cultures stimulated with soluble *Leishmania* antigen in patients with active lesions compared to individuals with subclinical disease. Ansari et al (2011) also associated active visceral leishmaniasis with elevated levels of IL-27 in plasma and IL-27 mRNA in spleen. IL-27 produced by macrophages, along with IL-21 from T cell sources, are suggested to be disease-promoting cytokines in visceral leishmaniasis by virtue of their roles in promoting the differentiation and expansion of Ag-specific, IL-10–producing T cells. The studies support the notion that IL-27 is a key instructional cytokine involved in regulating the balance between immunity and pathology in human visceral leishmaniasis [76].

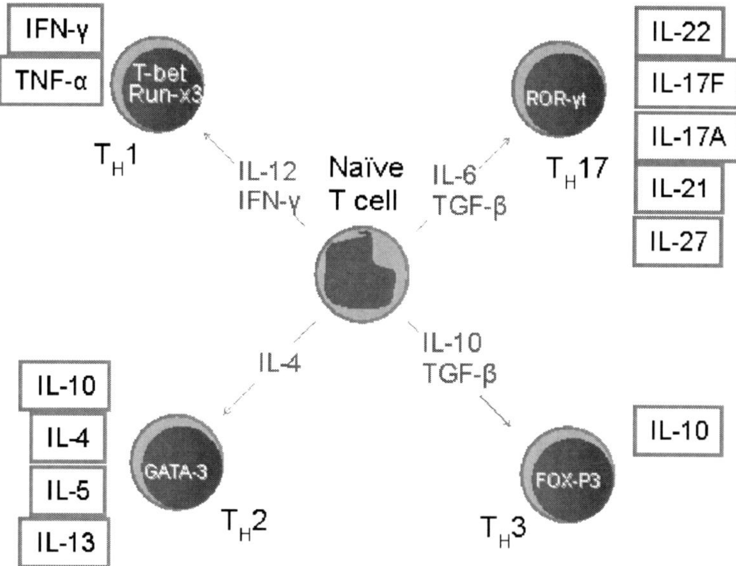

Figure 2. To all of the clinical forms of Leishmaniasis, the adaptive immune response is mainly executed by CD4$^+$ T-cells, through cytokine production. The development of a T cell profile may vary according the cytokine microenvironment. The presence of IFN-γ and IL-12 will contribute to set a Th1 profile, initially beneficial to the host, but harmful if exacerbated expressed. Th2 cells will dominate under influence of IL-4, which contributes to parasite growth and development of the disease. Cytokines such as IL-17A, IL17F and IL22 will be mainly secreted by Th17 cells, which develop in the presence of IL-6 and TGF-β. IL-27 works as a down-regulator of the profile. TGF-β is also required to the development of a regulatory response, mediated by IL-10 secretion by Foxp3$^+$ induced regulatory T cells.

3.4. Humoral Response

The infection by *Leishmania* in humans is characterized by the appearance of anti-leishmanial antibodies in the patients' serum. In respect of the humoral immune response, a successively high titer of specific antibodies can be observed in Localized ATL, Mucocutaneous Leishmaniasis (MCL) and Diffuse ATL. An exceptionally high titer of antibodies against *Leishmania* antigens can be detected in the most severe form of the disease, Visceral Leishmaniasis (VL), as a consequence of polyclonal activation of B cells resultant of the presence of large numbers of parasites in the bone marrow and spleen [79].

To evaluate the humoral immune response on Leishmaniasis, works have shown the role of the immunoglobulins on immunopathological mechanisms which are involved in the resistance and/or pathogenesis of the infection [80,81,82]. In some studies the presence of antibodies against *Leishmania braziliensis* in the sera of infected patients is still unclear but these antibodies have been monitored and they are utilized for diagnosis and prognosis of ATL [84,85]. Contrastingly, strong anti-leishmanial antibody titers are as well documented in VL [86,87].

However, it has been shown that the class IgG not only offers protection against this intracellular parasite, but indeed, it contributes to the progression of the infection. Previous analysis of *Leishmania* antigen-specific immunoglobulin isotypes and IgG subclasses in VL patients' sera has shown that elevated levels of IgG, IgM, IgE and IgG subclasses were lasting [79]. This is due to differential patterns of immunoglobulin isotypes observed during the disease progression. Drug resistance and cure were specific for antigens of *Leishmania donovani.* IgG subclass analysis has revealed expression of all the subclasses, with a prevalence of IgG1 during the disease [87], nevertheless, some studies have shown the advantage of using specific subclass antibodies for the diagnosis of VL [79,88,89].

Although studies have been evaluating the humoral immune response on ATL, the role of specific antibodies on the immunity against *Leishmania* is still not completely clear. On Cutaneous Leishmaniasis (CL) and Mucocutaneous Leishmaniasis (MCL), the cellular immunity and the prevalence of the isotypes IgG1, IgG2 and IgG3 have been associated with the Th1 response; on the other hand, the Th2 profile has been related to Diffuse Cutaneous Leishmaniasis (DCL), with the presence of IgG4. Studies lead the attention to the correlation of the subclasses of IgG with the clinical manifestations of ATL. Therefore, high levels of the isotypes IgG1, IgG2 and

IgG3 and low levels or absence of the IgG4 isotype can be detected in the sera of patients with CL. In patients with MCL, there are high levels of IgG1 while the levels of IgG2, IgG3 and IgG4 are similar to the findings on the sera of patients with CL. The levels of IgG4 in patients with DL are highly elevated, as the level of IgG1 and IgG2 are similar to the patients with CL and MCL. Studies show that all specific isotypes anti-*Leishmania,* except for IgD, are detected in the sera of patients with ATL. There are high levels of IgE in patients with more time of disease evolution and high levels of IgA in patients with MCL [82].

The intensity of the antibody response appears to reflect both the parasite load and the chronicity of the infection and it also can be observed high titers of antibodies in all clinical manifestations of ATL [90]. Studies with immunological and serological methods which are available to the research of antibodies in ATL, showed controversial results due to its low sensibility and specificity [91,92]. However, studies have shown the advantages of using specific antibodies in the diagnosis of VL [79,88,89].

4. Final Considerations

Classically, *Leishmania* infections can induce the host to mount an immune response, which is characterized by the enrichment of T CD4+ cells, with Th1 or Th2 cytokines profile. Although this definition exists, the complexity in host-parasite interaction has promoted the investigation of other response profiles, in which cytokines, molecules and mediators take part. These may contribute favorably or not in the evolution of the different clinical forms in leishmaniasis. The scientific community has evaluated distinct cell subtypes, such as regulatory T cells, that accumulate in the lesion site and also acts mediating immune response through effector cells. Recently the Th17 profile was evidenced, and it was firstly related to the pathogenesis of chronic inflammatory disease or autoimmunity. Furthermore, the involvement of antibodies in diagnostic evaluations and as a criterion of cure must be considered.

In the balance between cure and progress of the disease, studies have shown that regardless of the cell and or molecules of a given profile, none is sufficient to act independently in the immune response. Thus, the balance between the innate and adaptive immune system and the parasite evasion mechanisms is critical for the decision if disease is observed and if (lifelong) immunity develops [13].

REFERENCES

[1] Rogers, K. A. et al. 2002. Type 1 and type 2 responses to *Leishmania major*. *FEMS Microbiology Letters*, 209(1), 1-7.

[2] Brasil. (2007). Manual de Vigilância da leishmaniose tegumentar americana (2nd edition). Brasília, DF: Ministério da Saúde.

[3] Gontijo, B.; Carvalho, M. L. R. 2003. Leishmaniose Tegumentar Americana. *Rev. Soc. Bras. Med. Trop.*, 36 (1), 71-80.

[4] Birnbaum, R; Craft, N. (2011). Innate immunity and Leishmania vaccination strategies. *Dermatol. Clin. nina*, 29(1),89-102.

[5] Liese, J; Schleicher, U; Bogdan, C. (2008). The innate immune response against Leishmania parasites. *Immunobiology*, 213(3-4),377-87.

[6] Oghumu, S; Lezama-Dávila, CM; Isaac-Márquez, AP; Satoskar, AR. (2010).Role of chemokines in regulation of immunity against leishmaniasis. *Exp. Parasitol.,* 126(3),389-396.

[7] Faria, MS; Reis, FC; Lima, AP. (2012). Toll-like receptors in leishmania infections: guardians or promoters? *J. Parasitol. Res.*, 2012:930257, 12 pages.

[8] Kaye, P; Scott, P. (2011). Leishmaniasis: complexity at the host-pathogen interface. *Nat. Rev. Microbiol.*, 9(8), 604-615.

[9] Ritter, U; Frischknecht, F; van Zandbergen, G. (2009). Are neutrophils important host cells for Leishmania parasites? *Trends Parasitol.,* 25(11), 505-510.

[10] Peters, NC; Sacks, DL. (2009). The impact of vector-mediated neutrophil recruitment on cutaneous leishmaniasis. *Cellular Microbiology*, 11(9), 1290–1296.

[11] Nylén, S; Gautam, S. (2010) Immunological perspectives of leishmaniasis. *J. Glob. Infect. Dis.*, 2(2), 135-46.

[12] John, B; Hunter, CA. (2008). Neutrophil Soldiers or Trojan Horses? *Science*, 321, 917.

[13] Maurer, M; Dondji, B; Von Stebut, E. (2009). What determines the success or failure of intracellular cutaneous parasites? Lessons learned from leishmaniasis. *Med. Microbiol. Immunol.*, 198(3),137-146.

[14] Teixeira, MJ; Teixeira, CR; Andrade, BB; Barral-Netto, M; Barral, A. (2006). Chemokines in host-parasite interactions in leishmaniasis. *Trends Parasitol.*, 22(1), 32-40.

[15] Carvalho, LP; Pearce, EJ; Scott P. (2008). Functional dichotomy of dendritic cells following interaction with Leishmania braziliensis: infected cells produce high levels of TNF-alpha, whereas bystander

dendritic cells are activated to promote T cell responses. *J. Immunol.*, 181(9), 6473-80.

[16] Ritter, U; Körner, H. (2002). Divergent expression of inflammatory dermal chemokines in cutaneous leishmaniasis. *Parasite Immunol.*, 24(6), 295-301.

[17] Cummings, HE; Tuladhar, R; Satoskar, AR. (2010). Cytokines and their STATs in cutaneous and visceral leishmaniasis. *J. Biomed. Biotechnol.*, 2010, 294389, 6 pages.

[18] Bogdan, C. (2008). Mechanisms and consequences of persistence of intracellular pathogens: leishmaniasis as an example. *Cell Microbiol.*, 10(6),1221-1234.

[19] Srivastava, A; Singh, N; Mishra, M; Kumar, V; Gour, JK; Bajpai, S; Singh, S., Pandey, HP; Singh, RK. (2012). Identification of TLR inducing Th1-responsive Leishmania donovani amastigote-specific antigens. *Mol. Cell Biochem.*, 359(1-2),359-368.

[20] Baratta-Masini, A; Teixeira-Carvalho, A; Malaquias, LC; Mayrink, W; Martins-Filho, AO; Corrêa-Oliveira R. (2007). Mixed cytokine profile during active cutaneous leishmaniasis and in natural resistance. *Front Biosci.*, 12, 839-49.

[21] Kamali-Sarvestani, E; Rasouli, M; Mortazavi, H; Gharesi-Fard B. (2006). Cytokine gene polymorphisms and susceptibility to cutaneous leishmaniasis in Iranian patients. *Cytokine,* 35(3-4), 159-65.

[22] Singh, RK; Srivastava, A; Singh, N. (2012). Toll-like receptor signaling: a perspective to develop vaccine against leishmaniasis. *Microbiol. Res.*, 167(8),445-451.

[23] Rosas, L.E.; Keiser,T.; Barbi,J.; Satoskar,A.A.; Septer,A.; Kaczmarek,J.; Davila, C.M.L. and Satoskar, A.R.(2005). Genetic background influences immune responses and disease outcome of cutaneous L.mexicana infection in mice. *International. Immunology*, vol 17, pp 1347-1357.

[24] Cummings, H.E.; Tuladhar,R and Satoskar,A,R.(2010) Cytokines and their STATs in cutaneous and visceral Leishmaniasis. *Journal of biomedicine and biotechnology,* vol. 2010,6 pages.

[25] Sharma, U. and Singh, S. (2009). Immunobiology of leishmaniasis. *Indian Journal of Experimental Biology,* vol.47, pp 412-423.

[26] Mosmann,T.R.; Cherwinski,H., and Bond,M.W.(1986). Two types of murine helper T cell clone. I. Definition according to profiles of lymphokine activities and secreted proteins. *Journal of Immunology*, vol. 136, pp. 2348–2357.

[27] Horta, M.F.; Mendes,B.P.; Roma, E.H.; Noronha,F.S.M.; Macedo,J.P.; Oliveria,L.S.; Duarte,M.M. andVieira,L.Q. (2012). Reactive Oxygen Species and Nitric Oxide in Cutaneous Leishmaniasis. *Journal of Parasitology Research,* vol.2012,11 pages.

[28] Alexander, J.; Satoskar, A.R and Russell, D.G. (1999). Leishmania species: models of intracellular parasitism. *Journal of Cell Science*, vol.112, pp.2993-3002.

[29] Scott P. The role TH1 and TH2 cells in experimental cutaneous leishmaniasis.(1989). *Experimental Parasitology*, vol. 68, pp 369-372.

[30] Bogdan, C.; Rollinghoff, M. and Diefenbach, A. (2000). The role of nitric oxide in innate immunity. *Immunological Reviews*,vol.173.pp 17-26.

[31] Kedzierski L. (2010). Leishmaniasis Vaccine: Where Are We Today?. *Journal of Global Infectious Disease*, vol.2(2), 177–185.

[32] Stager, S.; Alexander,J.; Carter,K.C.; Brombacher,F. And Kaye, P.M. (2003) .Both Interleukin -4 (IL-4) and IL-4 receptor α signaling contribute to the development of hepatic granulomas with optimal antileishmanial activity. *Infection and Immunity*, vol.71. pp.4804-4807.

[33] Alexander, J.; Carter,K.C.; Al-Fasi,N.; Satoskar, A. and Brombacher, F. (2000). Endogenous IL-4 is necessary for effective drug therapy against visceral leishmaniasis. *European Journal of Immunology*, vol 30, pp. 2935-2943.

[34] Mocci, S. and Coffman,R.L.(1995). Induction of a Th2 population from a polarized Leshmania-specifc Th1 population by in vitro culture with IL-4. *The Journal of Immunology*, vol.154, pp.3779-3787.

[35] Sacks., D. and Noben-Trauth, N. (2002). The immunology of susceptibility and resistance to leishmania major in mice. *Nature Reviews Immunology*,vol.2(11),pp.845-58.

[36] Antonelli, L.R.V.; Dutra,W.O.; Almeida,R.P.; Bacellar,O. and Gollob, K.J. (2004). Antigen specific correlations of cellular immune responses in human leishmaniasis suggests mechanisms for immunoregulation. *Clinical and Experimental Immunology*, vol 136(2), pp.341-348.

[37] Liew, F.Y.; Xu, D. and Chan, W.L.(1999). Immune effector mechanism is parasitic infections. *Immunology Letters*, vol.65. pp.101-104.

[38] Chatelain, R.; Varkila, K. and Coffman, R.L.(1992). IL-4 induces a Th2 response in Leishmania major infected mice. *The Journal of Immunology,* vol.148, pp.1182-7.

[39] Wang, Z.E.; Reiner, S.L.; Zheng, S.; Dalton, D.K. and Locksley, R.M.(1994). CD4+ effector cells default to the Th2 pathway in

interferon gamma-deficient mice infected with Leishmania major.*The Journal of experimental Medicine,* vol.179, pp.1367-71.

[40] Chatelain, R.; Mauze, S. and Coffman, R.L.(1999).Experimental Leishmania major infection in mice: role of IL-10. *Parasite Immunology*, vol.21, pp.211-8.

[41] Harms, G.; Zwingenberger, K.; Chehade, A.K.; Talhari, S.; Racz, P.; Mouakeh, A.; Nakel,L.; Naiff,R.D.; and Kremsner,P.G. et al.(1989). Effects of intradermal gamma-interferon in cutaneous leishmaniasis. vol.1, pp.1287-92.

[42] Anderson, C.F.; Mendez, S. and Sacks DL. (2005). Nonhealing infection despite Th1 polarization produced by a strain of Leishmania major in C57BL/6 mice.*The Journal of Immunology*,vol.174. pp.2934-41.

[43] Sundar, S.; Rosenkaimer, F.; Lesser, M.L. and Murray, H.W. Immunochemotherapy for a systemic intracellular infection: accelerated response using interferon-gamma in visceral leishmaniasis. *The Journal of Infectious Diseases*, vol.171, pp.992-6.

[44] Nylen, S.; Khamesipour, A.; Mohammadi, A.; Jafari-Shakib, R.; Eidsmo, L. and Noazin, S. et al. (2006).Surrogate markers of immunity to Leishmania major in leishmanin skin test negative individuals from an endemic area re-visited. *Vaccine,*vol.24, pp.6944-54.

[45] Withie, C.; Debus, A.; Mohrs, M.; Steinkasserer, A.; Lutz, M. and Gessner, A.(2008). Dendritic cell differentiation state and their interaction with NKT cells determine Th1/Th2 differentiation in the murine model of Leishmania major infection. *Journal of Immunology,*vol. 180, pp.4371-4381.

[46] Belkaid, Y., Sun, C.M., Bouladoux, N., 2006b. Parasites and immunoregulatory T cells. *Curr. Opin. Immunol.*, 18, 406–412.

[47] Sakaguchi, S. et al. 1995. Immunologic self-tolerance maintained by activated T cells expressing IL-2 receptor alpha-chains (CD25). Breakdown of a single mechanism of self-tolerance causes various autoimmune diseases. *J. Immunol.*, 155, 1151–1164.

[48] Belkaid, Y., 2003. The role of CD4(+)CD25(+) regulatory T cells in *Leishmania infection. Exp. Opin. Biol. Th.*, 3, 875–885.

[49] Fontenot, J.D., Gavin, M.A., Rudensky, A.Y., 2003. Foxp3 programs the development and function of CD4+CD25+ regulatory T cells. *Nat. Immunol.*, 4, 330–336.

[50] Hori, S., Nomura, T., Sakaguchi, S., 2003. Control of regulatory T cell development by the transcription factor Foxp3. *Science,* 299, 1057–1061.

[51] Khattri, R., Cox, T., Yasayko, S.A., Ramsdell, F., 2003. An essential role for Scurfin in CD4+CD25+ T regulatory cells. *Nat. Immunol.*, 4, 337–342.

[52] Belkaid, Y. 2007. Regulatory T cells and infection: a dangerous necessity. *Nat. Rev. Immunol.*, 7(11), 875-88.

[53] Belkaid, Y., Piccirillo, C.A., Mendez, S., Shevach, E.M., Sacks, D.L., 2002. CD4+CD25+ regulatory T cells control *Leishmania major* persistence and immunity. *Nature*, 420, 502–507.

[54] Falcão, S. C. et al. 2012. The presence of Tregs does not preclude immunity to reinfection with *Leishmania braziliensis*. *Int. J. Parasitol.*, 42, 771–780.

[55] Campanelli A.P et al. 2006. CD4+CD25+ T cells in skin lesions of patients with cutaneous leishmaniasis exhibit phenotypic of natural regulatory T cells. *J. Infect. Dis.*, 193, 1313-1322.

[56] Piccirillo, C.A.; Thornton, A.M. 2004. Cornerstone of peripheral tolerance: naturally occurring CD4+CD25+ regulatory T cells. *Trends Immunol.*, 25:374–80.

[57] Read, S; Malmstrom, V; Powrie, F. 2000. Cytotoxic T lymphocyte-associated antigen 4 plays an essential role in the function of CD25+CD4+ regulatory cells that control intestinal inflammation. *J. Exp. Med.*, 192:295–302.

[58] Rai AK et al. 2012. Regulatory T Cells Suppress T Cell Activation at the Pathologic Site of Human Visceral Leishmaniasis. *Plos One* 7(2), 1-11.

[59] Nylen, S. et al. 2007. Splenic accumulation of IL-10 mRNA in T cells distinct from CD4+CD25+ (Foxp3) regulatory T cells in human visceral leishmaniasis. *J. Exp. Med.*, 204, 805–817.

[60] Almeida, A. F. et al. 2010. Immunophenotypic characterization of patients with American cutaneous leishmaniasis prior to and after treatment in Pernambuco, *Brazil. J. Venom. Anim. Toxins*, 17(2), 230-234.

[61] González-García, C. and Martín-Saavedra, F.M. and Ballester, A. and Ballester, S. (2009). The Th17 lineage: Answers to some immunological questions. *Inmunología,* 28(1): 32-45.

[62] Yao, Z. et al. (1995). Human IL-17: a novel cytokine derived from T cells. *J. Immunol.*, 155 (12):5483-5486.

[63] Schmidt-Weber, C. B. and Akdis, M. and Akdis, C. A. (2007). Th17 cells in the big picture of immunology. *Journal of Allergy and Clinical Immunology*, 120(2): 247-254.

[64] Oukka, M. (2007). Interplay between pathogenic Th17 and regulatory T cells. *Annals of the Rheumatic Diseases,* 66: 87-90.

[65] Torrado, E. and Cooper, A.M. (2010). IL-17 and Th17 cells in tuberculosis. *Cytokine Growth Factor Rev.,* 21(6):455-62.

[66] Guedes, P.M.M. et al. (2010). IL-17 Produced during Trypanosoma cruzi Infection Playsa Central Role in Regulating Parasite-InducedMyocarditis. *PLoS. Negl. Trop. Dis.*, 4(2):e604.

[67] Kaufmann SH, Kuchroo VK. 2009. Th17 cells. *Microbes Infect.,* 11(5):579-83.

[68] Kostka, S.L. et al. (2009). IL-17 Promotes Progression of Cutaneous Leishmaniasis in Susceptible Mice. *J. Immunol.*, 182:3039-3046.

[69] Happel, K.I. et al. (2003). Cutting Edge: Roles of Toll-Like Receptor 4 and IL-23 in IL-17 Expression in Response to Klebsiella pneumonia Infection. *J. Immunol.*, 170:4432-4436.

[70] Matsuzaki, G. and Umemura, M. (2007). Interleukin-17 as an effector molecule of innate and acquired immunity against infections. *Microbiology and Immunology*, 51(12):1139-1147.

[71] Kelly, M.N. et al. (2005). Interleukin-17/Interleukin-17 Receptor-Mediated Signaling Is Important for Generation of an Optimal Polymorphonuclear Response against Toxoplasma gondii Infection. *Infection and immunity*, 73(1): 617-621.

[72] Khader, S.A. and Gopal, R. (2010). IL-17 in protective immunity to intracellular pathogens. *Virulence,* 5(1):423-427.

[73] Rutitzky, L.I. and Lopes da Rosa, J.R. and Stadecker M.J. (2005). Severe CD4 T cell-mediated immunopathology in murine schistosomiasis is dependent on IL-12p40 and correlates with high levels of IL-17. *J. Immunol.,* 175: 3920–3906.

[74] Bacellar, O. et al. (2009). IL-17 Production in Patients with American Cutaneous Leishmaniasis. *J. Infect. Dis.,* 200(1): 75–78.

[75] Novoa, R. et al. (2011). IL-17 and Regulatory Cytokines (IL-10 and IL-27) in L. braziliensis Infection. *Parasite Immunol.*, 33(2): 132–136.

[76] Ansari, N.A. et al. (2011). IL-27 and IL-21 Are Associated with T Cell IL-10 Responses in Human Visceral Leishmaniasis. *J. Immunol.,* 186:3977-3985.

[77] Korn, T. and Bettelli, E. and Oukka, M. and Kuchroo, V.K. (2009). IL-17 and Th17 cells. *Annu. Rev. Immunol.*, 27:485–517.

[78] Pitta, M.G.R. et al. (2009). IL-17 and IL-22 are associated with protection against human kala azar caused by Leishmania donovani. *J. Clin. Invest.*, 119:2379–2387.

[79] Ozbilge, H; Aksoy, N; Gurel, MS; Yazar, S. (2006). IgG and IgG subclass antibodies in patients with active cutaneous leishmaniasis. *Journal of Medical Microbiology*, 55, 1329-1331.

[80] Rodriguez, V; Centeno, M; Ulrich, M. (1996). The IgG isotypes of specific antibodies in patients with American cutaneous leishmaniasis; relationship to the cell-mediated immune response. *Parasite Immunology*, 18(7), 341-345.

[81] Mosleh, IM; Saliba, EK; Al-Katheeb, MS; Bisharat, Z; Oumeish, OY; Bitar, W. (1995). Serodiagnosis of cutaneous leishmaniasis in Jordan using indirect antibody test and the enzyme-linked immunosorbent assay. *Acta Tropica*, 59, 163-172.

[82] O`Neil, CE; Labrada, M; Saraiva, NG. (1993). Leishmania (Viannia) panamensis – specific IgE and IgA antibodies relation to expression of human tegumentary leishmaniasis. The American *Journal of Tropical Medicine and Hygiene*, 49, 181-188.

[83] Rocha, RDR; Gontijo, CMF; Elói-Santos, SM; Carvalho, AT; Corrêa-Oliveira, R; Marques, MJ; Genaro, O; Mayrink, W; Martins-Filho, OA. (2002). Anticorpos antipromastigotas vivas de *Leishmania (Viannia) braziliensis*, detectados pela citometria de fluxo, para identificação da infecção ativa de leishmaniose tegumentar americana. *Revista da Sociedade Brasileira de Medicina Tropical,* 35, 551-562.

[84] Pissinate, JF; Gomes, IT; Peruhype-Magalhães, V; Dietze, R; Martins-Filho, OA; Lemos, EM. (2008). Upgrading the flow-cytometric analysis of anti-*Leishmania* immunoglobulins for the diagnosis of American tegumentary leishmaniasis. *Journal of Immunological Methods*, 336, 193-202.

[85] Neogy AB; Nandy A; Ghosh, DB; Chowdhury, AB. (1987). Antibody kinetics in kala-azar in response to treatment. *Annals of Tropical Medicine and Parasitology,* 81, 727-9.

[86] Saha, S; Mondal, S; Banerjee, A; Ghose, J; Bhowmick, S; Ali, N. (2006). Immune responses in kala-azar. *Indian Journal of Medical Research,* 123, 245-266.

[87] Anam, K; Afrin, F; Banerjee, D; Pramanik, N; Guha, SK; Goswami, RP; Gupta, PN; Saha, SK; Ali, N. (1999). Immunoglobulin subclass distribution and diagnostic value of Leishmania donovani antigen-specific immunoglobulin G3 in Indian kala-azar patients. *Clinical and Diagnostic Laboratory Immunology,* 6, 231–235.

[88] Chatterjee, M; Basu, K; Basu, D; Bannerjee, D; Pramanik, N; Guha, SK; Goswami, RP; Saha, SK; Mandal, C. (1998) Distribution of IgG

subclasses in antimonial unresponsive Indian kala-azar patients. *Clinical and Experimental Immunology*, 114(3), 408-413.

[89] Carvalho-Neta, A.V; Rocha, RDR; Gontijo, CMF; Reis, AB; Martins-Filho, OA. (2006). Citometria de fluxo no diagnóstico da leishmaniose visceral canina. *Arquivo Brasileiro de Medicina Veterinária e Zootecnia*, 58, 480-488.

[90] Trujillo, C; Ramirez, R; Vélez, ID; Berberich, C. (1999). The humoral immune response to the kinetoplastid membrane protein-11 in patients with American leishmaniasis and chagas disease: prevalence of IgG subclasses and mapping of epitopes. *Immunology Letters*, 70, 203-209.

[91] Ribeiro, FC; Schubach, AO; Mouta-Confort, E; Schubach, TMP; Madeira, MF; Marzochi, MCA. (2007). Use of ELISA employing Leishmania (Viannia) braziliensis and Leishmania (Leishmania) chagasi antigens for the detection of IgG and IgG1 and IgG2 subclasses in the diagnosis of American tegumentary leishmaniasis in dogs. *Veterinary Parasitology,* 148, 200-206.

[92] Boudoiseau, G; Hugnet, C; Gonçalves, RB; Vézilier, F; Petit-Didier, E; Papierok, G; Lemesre, JL. (2009). Effective humoral and cellular immunoprotective responses in Li ESAp-MDP vaccinated protected dogs. *Veterinary Immunology and Immunoparasitology*, 128, 71-78.

[93] Mohammadi, MR; Zeinali, M; Ardestani, SK; Karminia, A. (2006). Identification of novel Leishmania major antigens that elicit IgG2a response in resistant and susceptible mice. *Korean Journal of Parasitology,* 44(1), 43-48.

In: Leishmaniasis
Editor: Carlos Sepulveda

ISBN: 978-1-62417-700-2

Chapter 2

LEISHMANIASES: ETIOLOGY, EPIDEMIOLOGY AND CLINICAL HEMATOLOGY

Ernesto Vigna, Anna Grazia Recchia, Massimo Gentile, Sabrina Bossio, Laura De Stefano, Teresa Granata, Nadia Caruso, Maria Valeria Pellicanò, Stefania Franzese and Morabito Fortunato *

Unità Operativa Complessa di Ematologia,
Azienda Ospedaliera di Cosenza, Cosenza, Italy

ABSTRACT

Leishmaniasis occurs commonly in four continents and is considered to be endemic in 88 countries. Like many neglected diseases, leishmaniasis has a focal distribution and occurs in remote locations. It is a significant public-health problem, endemic in 88 countries, 72 of which are developing countries. In 2007, the Sixtieth World Health Assembly, WHO's decision-making body, adopted Resolution WHA60.13 regarding the control of leishmanaisis: it discusses the impact on disease-control issues, activities in the areas of screening, diagnosis and treatment, and

* Corresponding Author: Fortunato Morabito, MD. UOC Ematologia, Azienda Ospedaliera di Cosenza, viale della Repubblica snc, 87100 Cosenza, Italy. E-mail: fortunato_morabito@tin.it, Ph: +39-0984-681329, Fax: +39-0984-681329.

the search for more effective medicines, underlying factors of failure to control disease, including an update of epidemiological information. Recent WHO reports updating epidemiological data indicate that the core problem of leishmanaisis is the access to treatment. Here we focus our attention on reviewed epidemiology, clinical presentation, diagnosis and currentlyavailable treatment options.

Keywords: Leishmaniasis, epidemiology, treatment

1. INTRODUCTION

The leishmaniases are vector-borne diseases due to infection caused by parasitic protozoans belonging to the *Leishmania* genus (Kinetoplastida, Trypanosomatidae), which find hosts in various wild and domestic animals and can be occasionally transmitted to humans by insect vectors [1].

On May 2012 an epidemiological update based on the outcomes of WHO regional meetings, literature review and experts' opinion was made[2]. The report underlined that the core problem of leishmaniases eradication is access to treatment. These data represent the first update of the empirical database for leishmaniasis since 1991. A total of 98 countries and 3 territories across 5 continents reported endemic leishmaniasis transmission.Visceral and cutaneous leishmaniasis incidence ranges were estimated by country and epidemiological region based on reported incidence, underreporting rates, and the judgment of experts: approximately 0.2 to 0.4 cases and 0.7 to 1.2 million visceral leishmaniasis (VL) and cutaneous leishmaniasis (CL) cases, respectively, occur each year. More than 90% of global VL cases occur in India, Bangladesh, Sudan, South Sudan, Ethiopia and Brazil. About 30% of CL cases occur in the Americas, the Mediterranean basin and western Asia from the Middle East to Central Asia, while countries with the highest estimated case counts, Afghanistan, Algeria, Colombia, Brazil, Iran, Syria, Ethiopia, North Sudan, Costa Rica and Peru, together account for 70 to 75% of incidence. The global mortality from VL can only be estimated, because in many countries the disease is not reported or is frequently undiagnosed, especially where there is no access to medication. Mortality data were extremely sparse and were generally representedby hospital-based deaths only. However, community-based studies estimate case-fatality rates of more than 10% withan estimate of 20,000 to 40,000 leishmaniasis deaths per year [2].

Infection is more common in men than in women. Children aged 1–4 years are particularly at risk of infection in the Mediterranean regions, and childhood infection may account for more than half of all cases in some of these countries. [3-6] In the poorest communities VL is often associated with malnutrition, which is a symptom of more severe infection and a major risk factor for poorer clinical and treatment outcomes. [7-9] Ideally, in endemic areas both preventive nutritional programs for the general population as well as supplementary and therapeutic feeding interventions for VL patients should be in force since drug-dosing recommendations for VLtreatment are based on the patients' weight or age [10].

In the last 20 years, the epidemiology of leishmaniasis has been re-evaluated and interest in industrialized countries has increased due to the importance of travel medicine and also because of the inclusion of VL as a complication of HIV infection, with the result that theworldwide risk of infection estimate likely to be increased. [11]. Potential factors triggering changes in distribution areasmay include climate change, international travel, changes in environments (urbanisation,deforestation) and socio-economic patterns. [5, 11-14] Data about spatial distribution in Europe and the Mediterranean region are being enhanced and made accessible online by the EDEN project and the LeishRisk project. The EDEN leishmaniasis sub-project evidenced the necessityto cross human and veterinary data of disease notification for contention. [15-17] Epidemiological characteristics,apart from distribution, have also changed due to the appearance of HIV, with progressive increasing number of visceral cases observed in adults. HIV/Leishmaniaco-infections were recorded in 35 countries worldwide.[11] Recent *Leishmania* individuationin discarded syringes inferred widespread needle transmission of *L. infantum* in southwest Europe [18].

2. Transmission

There are at least 21 known*Leishmania* species worldwide that can cause cutaneous and/or visceral human leishmaniasis with most foci occurring in the tropics or subtropics.Natural transmission may be either zoonotic or anthroponotic, and is usually the result of the bite of a phlebotomine sandfly species (order Diptera, family Psychodidae; subfamily Phlebotominae) of the genera *Phlebotomus* (Old World) and *Lutzomyia* (New World), while the *L. donovan*i and *L. archibaldi*species cause periodic epidemics of anthroponotic VL ('Kala-azar') in India and northeast Africa, respectively. [19] In Europe only two transmission cycles have demonstrated long-term endemism:zoonotic visceral and cutaneous diseases caused by *L. infantum* throughout the Mediterranean region and sporadical anthroponotic cutaneous disease caused by *L. tropica* in Greece. *L. infantum* is transmitted in both the eastern and western hemispheres.[20] Prevalent transmission cycles are defined as zoonoses and involve reservoir hosts such as rodents, marsupials, edentates, monkeys, domestic dogs and wild canids; the domestic dog is the only reservoir host of major veterinary importance,but also domestic cats might be secondary reservoir hosts of *L. infantum* in Europe. [21-22] However Leishmaniasis can have anthroponotic transmission without the involvement of reservoir host (characteristic of species of the *L. tropica* complex and, except for *L. infantum*, of the *L. donovani* complex). Fortunately, vertical transmission of human Leishmania from mother to child has rarely been reported [23].

The life cycle of the parasitecan be distinguished by two morphological forms: flagellated promastigotes, which replicate and develop in the midgut of the sand-fly vector, and rounded amastigotes, which live and multiply inside the macrophages of the vertebrate host. The infective promastigote inoculated by the female sand-fly bite are phagocytised in the mammalian host by macrophages and related cells, in which it transforms to amastigote and multiplies. The amastigote proliferates in the mononuclear phagocyte system and produces disturbances in phagocyte bearing organs as well as haematological manifestations. In macrophages, amastigotes multiply inside the acidic vacuoles, and when released after lysisspread the infection to uninfected cells. A cutaneous lesion and ulcer at the site of the bite can be observed as a result of the immune reaction [24].

3. Clinical Manifestation

On the basis of clinical disease manifestations, human Leishmania infections are classified as visceral, cutaneous and mucocutaneous. Expression of the two basic forms depends on the species of *Leishmania* responsible and the immune response to infection. Primary skin infections (CL) heal spontaneously but leave scars, which, depending on the species of *Leishmania* responsible, may evolve into diffuse CL, recidivans leishmaniasis, or mucocutaneous leishmaniasis, with disastrous aesthetic consequences for the patient. The most severe form is VL and, is fatal in almost all cases if left untreated.

3.1. Cutaneous Disease

CL results from multiplication of Leishmania in the phagocytes of the skin by members of the L. mexicana complex (L. Mexicanamexicana, L. mexicana amazonensis, and L. Mexicanavenezuelensis) and the L. braziliensis complex (L. braziliensisbraziliensis, L. braziliensis panamensis, and L. braziliensis guyanensis) in the New World, and by L. tropica and L. major in the Old World [25].

After exposure,incubation period typically lasts from 2 weeks to several months, yet cases up to 3 years (Old World cutaneous Leishmaniasis) have been reported. First lesions appear as papules, at the site of a sand-fly bite, which then increases in sizesometimes with a nodular appearance and eventually progress to ulcers, which may take 3–18 months to heal with scarring. In New World CL, the incubation period is usually 2–8 weeks. In cases of disease due to *L. braziliensis,* lymphadenopathy may accompany the skin lesions or precede the skin lesions by 1-2 months.Leishmaniasis recidivans is characterised by tuberculoid lesions that are resistant to treatment which are localized around scars of healed cutaneous ulcers; lesions show a low parasite number on biopsy. This is more common in the New World Leishmania but also occurs with *L. aethiopica* in East Africa. In diffuse cutaneous disease, dissemination of skin lesions rarely occurs over the face, hands and feet, however when present they revealhigh parasite numbers due to poor cell-mediated immune response [26-28].

3.2. Mucosal Disease

Mucosal leishmaniasis by definition is an infection of the nose and mouth membranes. Initially presents in the nasal mucosa and then spreads to the oropharynx and larynx causing difficulty with eating and an increased risk of secondary infection which in turn carries a significant mortality. Mucosal involvement occurs in South American as a late sequel of New World cutaneous disease(espundia) or mucosal metastasis of the cutaneous lesion that does not heal spontaneously and evolves slowly (on average 3 years) before medical attention is sought. The incubation period is 1–3 months, although mucocutaneous leishmaniasis may occur many years after the initial cutaneous ulcer has healed [29].

3.3. Visceral Disease

Visceral disease (kala-azar) is the most severe form clinically. VLis primarily caused by *Leishmania donovani* in the Indian subcontinent and Africa, *Leishmania infantum* in Mediterranean regions, and *Leishmaniachagasi* in the New World; the latter two speciesare closely related [25]. The incubation period varies from 3 to 8 months (range 10 days to 34 months) [30] and may be asymptomatic and self-resolving. The disease usually runs a chronic course and may be fatal without or despite treatment, with death a consequence of severe secondary bacterial infections in advanced disease.

Clinical features of VL can be easily misinterpreted for other febrile illnesses such as malaria and enteric fever therefore reliable laboratory methods are required to establish an accurate diagnosis. Because the reticuloendothelial system is usually targeted, hepatosplenomegaly is a classical presentation.Further involvement of the haematological system occurs in peripheral blood and bone marrow and therefore makes differential diagnosis complicated in patients presenting with fever, hepato-splenomegaly, anaemia, and peripheral cytopenias (leukopenia, thrombocytopenia, and pancytopenia) or histiocytosis and disseminated intravascular coagulopathy (DIC) [30].

Other clinical manifestations include fever, and a peculiar grey discoloration of the skin of the hands, feet, abdomen and face—hence the common name ''kala azar,'' or ''black disease,'' given to the condition. Liver dysfunction may be caused directly by the protozoa or indirectly by the immune response of the parasites. Late stages may present with jaundice, ascitis and deranged coagulation and has a poor prognosis [28].

VL can also present atypically. Cases involving the lungs, pleura, oral mucosa, larynx, oesophagus, stomach, small intestine,neurological symptoms have been reported [27,31], as well as Guillain-Barre syndrome [32], leishmanial cholecystitis [33], acute renal injury [34], hepatitis [35], and congenital leishmaniasis [36]. In addition, monoclonal gammopathy and hormonal alteration have also been associated with VL [37,38].

Variants of VLhave been described: a mild variant of visceral disease that does not progress to classic kala-azar was described during Operation Desert Storm, as in that observed in Brazilian children who had high titres of antibodies to Leishmania, although completely asymptomatic or affected only bymild symptoms (malaise, diarrhoea, and poor tolerance of work or play) and intermittent hepatomegaly. [39] Likely, asymptomatic disease and mild disease are the most frequent forms of VL [40].

Post-kala azar dermal leishmaniasis (PKDL), a sequel of VL, is frequently observed in Sudan (Sudanese disease or "killing disease") and in the Indian subcontinent thatdevelops after resolution of VL. The time interval to development of PKDL is variable.This is usually due to infection by the *L. donovani sensu stricto* cluster.The skin lesions are macular, maculo-papular or nodular, and usually spread from the perioral area to other areas of the body, do not heal spontaneously but become denser and spread over the face, upper chest and back, upper arms, or over the entire body and included nodules and ulceration [41].

HIV-associated CL is rare. However, the coexistence of HIV and visceralizing Leishmania species in southern Europe and in a few other areas where leishmaniasis is endemichas resulted in a large number of dually infected individuals. The clinical presentation in HIV-infected hosts is comparable to the classic presentation with the notable exception of gastrointestinal tract involvement andhepatosplenomegaly [42] and CD4 cell counts relatively high [43].

3.4. Haematological Findings in Visceral Leishmaniasis

Since a variable degree of frequency and severity of pancytopenia has been reported by several patient settings, this calls for a differential diagnosis with haematological diseases.When pancytopenia is associated with fever, hepatosplenomegaly and lymphadenopathy, bone marrow examination easily differentiates VL from leukaemia or lymphoma.Normochromic normocytic anaemia is frequent with multifactorial causes [44]: haemolysis with little evidence of ineffective erythropoiesis and hypersplenism are major causes due to the sequestration red blood cells in the enlarged spleen and the lysis of recruited macrophages to the spleen and liver as part of inflammatory response. [45] Reticuloendothelial hyperplasia is accompanied by abnormal iron retention by macrophages, and may limit the marrow response to haemolysis. [46] In most cases there is no evidence of immune haemolysishowever the immune response and alterations in membrane cell permeability due to increased sensitivity to complement, inhibition of erythrocyte enzymes, production of haemolysin by the parasites and presence of cold agglutinins may play a contributory role [30].

Leukopenia is often present and is a main resultof hypersplenism. The relative lymphocytosis with neutropenia, with absence of eosinophils and the presence of significant numbers of eosinophils rules out the diagnosis of VL. A change in platelet counts are usually affected after prolonged illness and is alsoattributable to splenic sequestration. [47] Platelet function studies reported reduction of platelet adhesive index and abnormal platelet aggregation time, with ADP and adrenaline similar to controls in a variable percentage of patients [48].

Splenic sequestration, ineffective haematopoiesis and hemophagocytosis appear to be the main etiopathogenetic factors in the emergence of hypercellular marrow with peripheral cytopenias but there is no significant correlation with degree of parasitemia. [49] Reversal in myeloid erythroid ratio and mild to moderate dyserythropoiesis is frequentlypresent. [50] Most common findings include erythroid hyperplasia with moderate to severe megaloblastosis, deficient iron stores or features of dual deficiency, increased plasma cells and intracellular parasites in mononuclear phagocytes with no alteration in granulocytic or megakaryocyte morphology. [51] Histiocytic hyperplasia produces syncytium like arrangement on bone marrow examination. Hemophagocytosis has been observed as a common morphological finding along with variable degrees of granulomatous reaction and marrow necrotizing granulomas in patients with VL have been shown to be associated with poor prognosis.Also common is an increased vessel density leading to neoangiogenesis, possibly linked to the release of cytokines secondary to infection [52-53].

4. Diagnostic Methods

Criteria for diagnosis of leishmaniasis are based on epidemiological data, clinical features and laboratory test results. Demonstration of the parasites in stained preparations (splenic and bone marrow aspirate) is still the gold standard for VL diagnosis but serological studies are recommended as the initial diagnostic tests in suspected leishmaniasis.

The serological diagnosis is based on the presence of specific humoral response. A wide range of serological methods varying in sensitivity and specificity are available for the diagnosis of VL.

The direct agglutination test (DAT) can easily detect high serological titresand represents a good option in endemic areas to confirm diagnosis in patients presenting suggestive symptoms. DAT is able to detect low levels of antibodies due to the mosaic of antigens present in the extract, but has limited success due to the variability in the techniques and preservation of the antigen and high levels of cross reactivity with other trypanosomatides [54].

Third generation tests for the sierodiagnosis of VL have utilized combinations of enzyme-linked immunosorbent assay (ELISA) and immunochromatography. A recent meta-analysis comparing different sierodiagnositic tests of VL currently available [55] showed that the rK39 protein used either in a strip test or in an ELISA, and the DAT are the best choices for rapid and efficient sierodiagnosis.Maia et al. suggest using both rK39 strip test and DAT prior to initiating anti-Leishmania treatment when demonstration of the parasite in bone marrow or spleen aspirate biopsies is not available.

Antibody detection tests should complement other diagnostic tests like the hypersensitivity Montenegro reaction (leishmanin skin test); however the latter is limited to the detection of past infection and inapplicable during active disease due to complete anergy of the patient [56].

In advance stages of the disease, parasites can be diagnosed in the histopathology laboratory by direct visualization of the amastigotes. Aspirates of infected muco-cutaneous tissue and aspirates or biopsy specimens of involved visceral tissues (e.g., the spleen, liver, or bone marrow) are similarly subjected to microscopic examination and culture. Amastigotes can bepresent within monocytes or, less commonly, in neutrophils in the peripheral blood and in macrophages in bone marrow aspirates on slides stained with Leishman or Giemsa as small, round bodies 2–4 μm in diameter with indistinct cytoplasm, a nucleus, and a small rod-shaped kinetoplast. Extracellular free lying Leishmania donovani bodies (LD bodies)may also be seen from the disrupted cells [54].

Culture of bone marrow is, however, a more sensitive diagnostic technique than microscopy. Aspirates are collected aseptically and cultured in Novy–MacNeal–Nicolle medium or in Schneiders Drosophilia medium supplemented with calf serum. In 2–5 days, cultures usually begin to show promastigotes. Generally however, both staining and culture should be performed [57].

Most diagnoses are only genus-specific, being based on symptoms, the microscopic identification of parasites in Giemsa-stained smears of tissue or fluid, and serology. [56] The gold standard to identify *Leishmania* species and strains is multi-locus enzyme electrophoresis (MLEE) but more practical is to identify the isoenzyme strains (or zymodemes) by directly characterising the enzyme genes. [58] In addition, PCR of the internal transcribed spacer of the multi-copy nuclear ribosomal genes is the most common molecular technique successfully used for diagnosis and differentiation of species. [59-60] Monoclonal antibodies are not widely used but are available for the identification species and serotyping [61].

5. Treatment

Pentavalent Antimony

The National Kala-Azar Elimination Programmewas established in 2005 in India, Nepal and Bangladesh to reduce disease prevalence by 20- to 30-fold to less than 1/10,000 population by 2015. [62] Recommended first-line therapy treatment of cutaneous and VL by the WHO consists of an organic salt, pentavalent antimony, at dose of 20 mg/kg/die given daily intravenously (i.v.) or intramuscularly (i.m.) for 20-28 consecutive days. [63] Organic salts of pentavalent antimony act by inhibiting the enzymes of glycolysis and other metabolic pathways. [64] A maximum dose of 850 mg daily has been recommended in order to minimise side effects (fatigue, body-ache, electro-cardiographic abnormalities, elevated aminotransferase levels and chemical pancreatitis). Arecent randomised trial in US military personnel showed a shorter, 10-day course to be equally effective. [65] A novel liposome-based meglumine antimoniate formulation also appears to be promising [66].

The clinical response to antimonies is very rapid in cutaneous leishmaniasis, while in VL, fever reduction requires approximately four days, while splenomegaly reduces after only a few weeks. Recurrences are observed in a few immunocompetent patients, but almost in 100% of immuno-compromised patients [67].

Pentavalent antimony resistance is increasing and is a major problem particularly in North Bihar, India, where the failure rate for this treatment is greater than 50% [68].

Pentamidine/Diamidine

Pentamidine isothienate (4 mg/kg i.m., thrice-weekly for six weeks) can be used in treatment-resistant cases of VL. Its use is limited by its toxicity (myalgia, nausea, headache and hypoglycaemia, risk of irreversible diabetes), necessitating close inpatient monitoring. [69] Besides, pentamidine has poor response rates when used as a second-line drug in antimonial-resistant areas [70].

Paromomycin

Paromomycin (aminosidine) is an aminoglycosidic antibiotic active when used alone, however when combined with antimonials (12-18mg/kg i.m., daily for 21 days) it allows a reduction in the duration of the therapy. [71] It is cheaper and well-tolerated [72] and may be more efficient than antimonials alonein areas with high levels of antimonial resistance [73].

Miltefosine

Hexadecylphosphocholine (miltefosine) is the first effective orally active drug againstleishmaniasis. It is an alkylphosphocholine but its mechanisms of action against Leishmania have not yet been well defined: it has been shown to block the proliferation of Leishmania and to alter phospholipid and sterol composition [74] with no direct cytotoxic effects on the parasite, but with activation of host cellular immunity [75].

Dosing 2.5mg/kg/day over days 21-28 days appeared efficient both in untreated VL and in antimony-resistant VL (cure rate of 95–100%). [76] Miltefosinehas a very good safety profile: vomiting and diarrhoea are the most frequent side effects. Of note, miltefosine has toxic effects on reproductive capacity in female animals, and pregnancy should be strictly avoided while on therapy and for the following two months after therapy completion. When compared with amphotericin B in 6-month follow-up studies, respectively, the cure rates were 94% *versus* 97%. [76] Using intention-to-treat analysis, the cure rate in a Phase IV outpatient study in Bihar was only 82%. [77] However, miltefosine is considered most expensive.

Amphotericin B and Lipid-Associated Formulations

Amphotericin B probably intercalates with the parasite episterol precursors of ergosterol. It is used frequently in VL treatment and currently represents a well-established alternative first-line therapy for leishmaniasis. The trend in Southern Europe is shifting towards using liposome-associated amphotericin B (AmBL) as first-line treatment, even though the response rate is approximately 90% for antimonials. However, a recent trend in increasing resistance to pentavalent antimonials in this area has been recorded, possibly attributed to the useof meglumine antimonate to treat infected dogs [78].

Amphotericin B Desoxycholate (Fungizone®) showed 98% long-term cure in both antimonial-unresponsive and previously untreated patients [79]. Short-course treatment with amphotericin B-fat emulsion (five alternate-day infusions of 2 mg/kg) has been evaluated in an uncontrolled study in India with a reported cure rate of 93% in antimonial-unresponsive patients: this could represent a cost-effective treatment for patients with VL, including those with antimonial-unresponsive infection [80].

The alternative is to use one of three liposomal formulations available, Ambisome®(liposomal formulation using spherical, unilamellar particle), Amphocil®(cholesterol sulfate dispersion formulation), Abelcet® (ribbon-like lipid structure using a phospholipid matrix), which are highly effective and less toxic but more expensive.There are regional differences in responsiveness to the lipid formulations and in HIV-co-infected patients and in recipients of organ transplants; higher dosages and prolonged treatment are needed.

AmBL was highly acceptable and without toxicity in daily dosage regimens of 2-4 mg/kg i.v. in trial treatments of VL due to *Leishmania Infantum*. A non-randomized and multicentre clinical study showed nearly 100% efficacy, with a total dose of approximately 20 mg of AmBL/kg subdivided in six courses over 10 days. [81] Instead, amphotericin B colloidal dispersion, demonstrated a high efficacy with low dosage of 2 mg/kg i.v. for 5-7 days. Nevertheless, unlike AmBL, this compound revealed to be moderately toxic [82,83]. Amphotericin B lipid complex has been used with a dosage of 3 mg/kg/die i.v. for 5 days for the therapy of VL unresponsive to antimony in Indian patients: although anti-parasitic activity resulted excellent (100% recovery), collateral effects are of a certain entity. [84] The effectiveness of short courses of this liposomal amphotericin B has resulted in improved cost-benefits. [85,86] Studies using lower doses of this agent are also showing promise to improve cost-effective treatment in resource poor areas with high antimonial resistance [87].

Other Drugs

Numerous oral agents have been tested as stand-alone agents or as agents for combination therapy for treatment of VL. The imidazole and triazole drugs are not recommended for use in VL,however oral fluconazole and has been found useful in *L. major* infections, with a cure rate of 79%.Ketoconazole has been studied in *L. braziliensis panamensis* with efficacy (74%) similar to that of stibogluconate (68%).

Imiquimod, a topical immunomodulator has been successfully used in combination with meglumine antimonate in cutaneus cases resistant to meglumine alone [88].

Sitamaquine (WR6026), when administered to 1 mg/kg/day for 4 weeks provided a 50% cure rate. [89] More recently, a phase 2 dose-escalating trial was performed in Brazil. Cure rates for patients treated for 28 days were 0% and 67% at 1 mg/kg/day and 2 mg/kg/day, respectively. [90,91] Further studies are needed to determine the efficacy and toxicity profile of this agent.

Interferon gamma alone has limited efficacy in human VL. [92] Association treatment improves the response to antimonial therapy in some difficult cases, but the high cost of interferon gamma precludes its widespread use in the developing world.

Table 1. Available treatment options in leishmaniasis

Treatment	Dose
Pentavalent Antimony.	20 mg/kg/die given daily intravenously (i.v.) or intramuscularly (i.m.) for 20-28 consecutive days
Pentamidine/Diamidine	4 mg/kg im, thrice- weekly for six weeks
Paromomycin	12-18mg/kg for 21 days
Miltefosine (Hexadecylphosphocholine)	Dosing 2.5mg/kg/day over 21-28 days
Amphotericin B and Lipid-associated Formulations or Amphotericin B Desoxycholate	2-4 mg/kg i.v.

CONCLUSION

Although there have been great achievements with the existing tools, there is a definite need forcontinued investment in diagnostics, treatment andprevention of Leishmaniasis particularly in poorer countries. The development of the rK39 diagnostic test has allowed the rapid primary diagnosis, butfurther test development and evaluation is required, with specific attention to the diagnosticaccuracy in HIV co-infected patients and for the diagnosisof relapses and to assess treatment efficacy. Further investmentin immunochemotherapydeserves further attention.

More importantly, thedevelopment of improved therapies and a better understanding of parasite lifecycle should be accompanied by the development of methods to monitor drug resistance.

Finally, an effectivevaccine would significantly improve control of CL and particularly of VL, since the simple nature of the parasite lifecycle and the fact that healing and recovery protects individuals from reinfection indicate that it should be possible to develop a vaccine against VL.[93] Moreover, new methods to control the animal reservoirin *L. infantum*-endemic areas (for example dog collars)or to prevent human infection (such as insecticide impregnated bednets or blankets) will help to eradicate or effectively reduce exposure to the parasite.

It is only through the translation of the extensive knowledge of leishmanial biology into more effective diagnostic, treatment and prevention tools are essential steps to remove CL and VL from thelist endemic diseases. More importantly, suchefforts will be efficacious only if these tools areavailable to all patients regardless of economic status. Therefore there is an urgent need for sustainedcommitment for the eradication of this disease.

Acknowledgments

We thank Fondazione ‘Amelia Scorza’ onlus, Cosenza, Italy. We thank Brigida Gulino for precious secretarial assistance.

References

[1] Herwaldt, BL. Leishmaniasis. *Lancet,* 1999 354, 1191–1199.

[2] World Health Organization (WHO). Leishmaniasis: worldwide epidemiological and drug access update. *World Health Organ Tech Rep Ser*. 2012 [cited 2012 Oct 22]. Available from:http://www.who.it/entity /leishmaniasis.

[3] Guerin, PJ; Olliaro, P; Sundar, S; Boelaert, M; Croft, SL; Desjeux, P; Wasunna, MK; Bryceson, AD. Visceral leishmaniasis: current status of control, diagnosis, treatment and a proposed research and development agenda. *Lancet Infect Dis.,* 2002 2, 494 – 501.

[4] Camargo, LB; Langoni, H. Impact of leishmaniasis on public health. *Trop Dis.*, 2006 12, 527–548.

[5] Desjeux, P. The increase in risk factors of leishmaniasis worldwide. *Trans R. Soc. Trop. Med. Hyg.*, 2001 95:239-43

[6] Grech, V; Mizzi, J; Mangion, M; Vella, C. Visceral leishmaniasis in Malta—an 18 year paediatric, population based study. *Arch. Dis. Child,* 2000 82, 381–5.

[7] Anstead, GM; Chandrasekar, B; Zhao, W; Yang, J; Perez, LE; Melby, PC. Malnutrition alters the innate immune response and increases early visceralization following Leishmania donovani infection. *Infect Immun.*, 2001 69, 4709–4718.

[8] Malafaia, G. Protein-energy malnutrition as a risk factor for visceral leishmaniasis: a review. *Parasite Immunol.* 2009 31, 587–596.

[9] Mueller, Y; Mbulamberi, DB; Odermatt, P; Hoffmann, A; Loutan, L; Chappuis, F. Risk factors for in-hospital mortality of visceral leishmaniasis patients in eastern Uganda. *Trop. Med. Int. Health*, 2009 14, 910–917.

[10] Harhay, MO; Olliaro, PL; Vaillant, M; Chappuis, F; Lima, MA; Ritmeijer, K; Costa, CH; Costa, DL; Rijal, S; Sundar, S; and Balasegaram, M. Who is a typical patient with Visceral Leishmaniasis? Characterizing the demographic and nutritional profile of patients in Brazil, East Africa, and South Asia, *Am. J. Trop. Med. Hyg.*, 2011 84(4), 543–550.

[11] Desjeux, P; Alvar, J. Leishmania/HIV co-infections: epidemiology in Europe. *Ann. Trop. Med. Parasitol.* 2003 97, Suppl 1:3-15.

[12] Kuhn, KG. Global warming and leishmaniasis in Italy. *Bull Trop. Med. Int. Health,* 1999 7, 1–2.

[13] Martinez, S; Vanwambeke, SO; Ready, P. Linking changes in landscape composition and configuration with sandfly occurrence in southwest France. Fourth International Workshop on the Analysis of Multi-temporal Remote Sensing Images, 2007. MultiTemp.

[14] Ready, PD. Leishmaniasis emergence and climate change. In: S de la Roque, editor. Climate change: the impact on the epidemiology and control of animal diseases. *Rev. Sci. Tech. Off Int. Epiz,* 2008 27(2), 399-412.

[15] Dujardin, JC; Campino, L; Cañavate, C; Dedet, JP; Gradoni, L; Soteriadou, K; Mazeris, A; Ozbel, Y; Boelaert M. Spread of vector-borne diseases and neglect of Leishmaniasis, Europe. *Emerg. Infect Dis.*, 2008 14(7), 1013-8.

[16] LeishRisk [Internet]. Belgium: European Commission. [cited 2009 Mar 16]. Available from: http://www.leishrisk.net.
[17] World Organisation for Animal Health (OIE). OIE Listed diseases. France: OIE. [cited 2012 Oct 22]. Available from: http://www.oie.int /en/animal-health-in-the-world/oie-listed-diseases-2012/.
[18] Cruz, I; Morales, MA; Noguer, I; Rodríquez, A; Alvar, J. Leishmania in discarded syringes from intravenous drug users. *Lancet.* 2002 359(9312),1124-5.
[19] Killick-Kendrick, R. Phlebotomine vectors of the leishmaniases: a review. *Med. Vet. Entomol.,* 1990 4(1), 1-24.
[20] Sharma, U; Singh, S. Insect vectors of Leishmania: distribution, physiology and their control. *J. Vector Borne Dis.,* 2008 45, 255–272.
[21] Trotz-Williams, LA; Trees, AJ. Systematic review of the distribution of the major vector-borne parasitic infections in dogs and cats in Europe. *Vet. Rec.,* 2003 152(4), 97-105.
[22] World Health Organization. Control of the Leishmaniases. Report of a WHO Expert Committee. *World Health Organ Tech. Rep. Ser.,* 1990 793, 1-158.
[23] Meinecke, CK; Schottelius, J; Oskam, L; Fleischer, B. Congenital transmission of visceral leishmaniasis (Kala Azar) from an asymptomatic mother to her child. *Pediatrics,* 1999 104(5), e65.
[24] Kaye, P, Scot, P, Leishmaniasis: complexity at the hostpathogen interface. *Nature Reviews Microbiology*, 2011 9(8), 604–615.
[25] Grimaldi, G, Jr; Tesh, RB; McMahon-Pratt, D. A review of the geographic distribution and epidemiology of leishmaniasis in the new world. *Am. J. Trop. Med. Hyg,* 1989 41, 687-725.
[26] Herwaldt, BL; Arana, BA; Navin, TR. The natural history of cutaneous leishmaniasis in Guatemala. *J. Infect Dis.,* 1992165, 518-27.
[27] Mandell, GL; Bennett, JE; Mandell, DR, Douglas and Bennett's principles and practice of infectious diseases, 6th ed. Philadelphia, PA: Elsevier Churchill Livingstone, 2005 2428–42.
[28] Manson-Bahr, PEC, Apted FIC. Leishmaniasis. In: Manson-Bahr PEC, Apted FIC, eds. Manson's tropical diseases, 18th ed. London: Bailliere Tindall, 1982 93–115.
[29] Marsden, PD; Nonata, RR. Mucocutaneous leishmaniasis—a review of clinical aspects. *Rev. Soc. Bras Med. Trop.,* 1975 9, 309–26.
[30] Varma, N; Naseem, S, Hematologic Changes in Visceral Leishmaniasis/Kala Azar. *Indian J. Hematol. Blood Transfus,* 2010, 26(3), 78–82.

[31] Hashim, FA; Ahmed, AE; el-Hassan, M; el Mubarak, MH; Yagi, H; Ibrahim EN; Ali, MS. Neurologic changes in visceral leishmaniasis. *Am. J. Trop. Med. Hyg.,*199552,149-.

[32] Fasanaro, AM; Scoleri, G; Pizza, V; Gaeta, GB; Fasanaro, A. Guillain-Barre syndrome as presenting manifestation of visceral leishmaniasis [letter]. *Lancet,* 1991, 338-1142.

[33] Fahal, AH; El-Hag, IA; El-Hassan, AM; Hashim, FA. Leishmanial cholecystitis and colitis in a patient with visceral leishmaniasis. *Trans R Soc. Trop. Med. Hyg,* 1995, 89-284.

[34] Oliveira, MJ; Silva Júnior, GB; Abreu, K; Rocha, NA; Garcia, AV; Franco, LF; Mota,RM; Libório, AB; Daher, EF. Risk Factors for Acute Kidney Injury in Visceral Leishmaniasis (Kala-Azar). *Am. J. Trop. Med. Hyg.*, 2010 82(3),449–453

[35] Hervas, JA; Alberti, P; Ferragut, J; Canet, R. Acute hepatitis as a presenting manifestation of kala-azar. *Pediatr Infect Dis. J.,* 199 110, 409-10.

[36] Eltoum, IA; Zijlstra, EE; Ali, MS; Ghalib, HW; Satti, MM; Eltoum, B; el-Hassan, AM. Congenital kala-azar and leishmaniasis in the placenta. *Am. J. Trop. Med. Hyg,*199246,57-62.

[37] Vishal, Sharma et al. Monoclonal gammopathy associated with visceral leishmaniasis. *Braz. J. Infect Dis.* 2010 14(3),297-298.

[38] Verde, FA; Verde, FA; Neto, AS; Almeida, PC; Verde, EM. Hormonal disturbances in visceral leishmaniasis (kala-azar). *Am. J. Trop. Med. Hyg.,* 2011 84(5),668-73.

[39] Magill, AJ; Grogl, M; Johnson, SC; Gasser, RA Jr. Visceral infection due to Leishmania tropica in a veteran of Operation Desert Storm who presented 2 years after leaving Saudi Arabia [letter]. *Clin. Infect Dis.* 1994 19, 805-6.

[40] Badaro, R; Jones, TC; Carvalho, EM; Sampaio, D; Reed, SG; Barral, A; Teixeira, R; Johnson, WD Jr. New perspectives on a subclinical form of visceral leishmaniasis. *J. Infect Dis.* 1986 154,1003-11.

[41] Zijlstra, EE; El-Hassan, AM. Post kala-azar dermal leishmaniasis. *Trans R Soc Trop. Med. Hyg.,* 2001 95(Supp 1), S59–76.

[42] Rosenthal, E; Marty, P; Poizot-Martin, I et al. Visceral leishmaniasis and HIV-1 co-infection in southern France. *Trans. R. Soc. Trop. Med. Hyg.,* 1995 89,159-62.

[43] Altos, J; Salas, A; Riera, M et al. Visceral leishmaniasis: another HIVassociated opportunistic infection? Report of eight cases and review of the literature. *AIDS* 1991 5, 201-7.

[44] Kasli, EG. Hematological abnormalities in visceral leishmaniasis. *East Afr. Med. J.,* 1980 57,634–640.

[45] Woodroff, AW; Topley, E; Knight, R; Downie, CGB. The anaemia of kala-azar. *Br. J. Hematol.,* 1972 22, 319–329.

[46] Pippard, MJ; Moir, D; Weatherall, DJ;Lenicker, HM. Mechanism of anaemia in resistant visceral leishmaniasis. *Ann. Trop. Med. Parasitol.,* 1986 80 (3), 317-23.

[47] al-Jurayyan, NA; al-Nasser, MN; al-Fawaz, IM; al Ayed, IH; al Herbish, AS; al-Mazrou, AM; al Sohaibani, MO. The haematological manifestations of visceral leishmaniasis in infancy and childhood. *J. Trop. Pediatr,* 1995 41(3),143-8.

[48] Dube, B; Arora, A; Singh, VP; Kumar, K; Sunder, S. Platelet function studies in Indian kala-azar. *J. Trop. Med. Hyg.*, 1995 98(3),166-68.

[49] Calvo, JM; Hernández, JM; Palencia, J; Sierra, E. Visceral leishmaniasis presenting with peripheral leukocytosis and lymphocytosis. *Sangre (Barc).* 1994 39(1),57-8. Spanish.

[50] Sheikha, A. Dyserythropoiesis in 105 patients with visceral leishmaniasis. *Lab. Hematol.*, 2004 10(4), 206-11.

[51] Bhatia, P; Haldar, D; Varma, N; Marwaha, R; Varma, S. A case series highlighting the relative frequencies of the common, uncommon and typical/unusual hematological findings on bone marrow examination in cases of visceral leishmaniasis. *Mediterr J. Hematol. Infect Dis.*, 2011 3(1), e2011035.

[52] Kumar, PV; Vasei, M; Sadeghipour, A; Sadeghi, E; Soleimanpour, H; Mousavi, A; Tabatabaei, AH; Rizvi, MM. Visceral leishmaniasis: bone marrow biopsy findings. *J. Pediatr Hematol. Oncol.*, 2007 29(2),77-80.

[53] Horst, AK; Bickert, T; Brewig, N; Ludewig, P; van Rooijen, N; Schumacher, U; Beauchemin N; Ito, WD; Fleischer, B; Wagener, C; Ritter, U. CEACAM1+ myeloid cells control angiogenesis in inflammation. *Blood.* 2009 113(26), 6726-36.

[54] Srivastava, P; Dayama, A; Mehrotra, S;Sundar, Shyam . Diagnosis of visceral leishmaniasis. *Trans. R. Soc. Trop. Med. Hyg.*, 2011 105(1), 1–6.

[55] Maia, Z; Lírio, M; Mistro, S; Mendes, CM; Mehta, SR; Badaro, R. Comparative study of rK39 Leishmania antigen for serodiagnosis of visceral leishmaniasis: systematic review with meta-analysis. *PLoS Negl. Trop. Dis.,* 2012 6(1), e1484.

[56] World Organisation for Animal Health (OIE). Manual of Diagnostic Tests and Vaccines for Terrestrial Animals. OIE. 2012. [cited 2012 Oct

23]. Available from: http://www.oie.int/en/international-standard-setting/terrestrial-manual/access-online/.

[57] Navin, TR; Arana, FE; de Merida, AM; Arana, BA; Castillo, AL; Silvers, DN. Cutaneous leishmaniasis in Guatemala: comparison of diagnostic methods. *Am. J. Trop. Med. Hyg.* 1990 42,36-42.

[58] Zijlstra, EE; El-Hassan, AM. Visceral leishmaniasis. *Trans. R. Soc. Trop. Med. Hyg.*, 2001 95(Suppl 1), S27–58.

[59] Alvar, J; Barker, JR. Molecular tools for epidemiological studies and diagnosis of leishmaniasis and selected other parasitic diseases. *Trans. R. Soc. Trop. Med. Hyg.*, 2002 96,1-250.

[60] Salotra, P; Sreenivas, G; Pogue, GP; Lee, N; Nakhasi, HL; Ramesh, V; Negi, NS. Development of a species-specific PCR assay for detection of Leishmania donovani in clinical samples from patients with kala-azar and post-kala-azar dermal leishmaniasis. *J. Clin. Microbiol.,* 2001 39, 849–54.

[61] Ardehali, S; Moattari, A; Hatam, GR; Hosseini, SM; Sharifi, I. Characterization of Leishmania isolated in Iran: 1. Serotyping with species specific monoclonal antibodies. *Acta Trop.*, 2000 75(3), 301-7.

[62] Mondal, D; Singh, SP; Kumar, N etal. Visceral leishmaniasis elimination programme in India, Bangladesh, and Nepal: reshaping the case finding/case management strategy. *PLoS Negl. Trop.,* 2009Dis.3, e35.

[63] Gradoni, L; Bryceson, A; Desjeux, P. Treatment of Mediterranean visceral leishmaniasis. *Bull. World Health Organ*, 1995 73, 191–197.

[64] Berman, JD. Chemotherapy for leishmaniasis: biochemical mechanisms, clinical efficacy, and future strategies. *Rev. Infec Dis.,* 1988 10, 560-86.

[65] Wortmann, G; Miller, RS; Oster, C, et al. A randomized, double-blind study of the efficacy of a 10- or 20-day course of sodium stibogluconate for treatment of cutaneous leishmaniasis in United States military personnel. *Clin. Infect Dis.,* 2002 35, 261–7.

[66] Frezard, F; Michalick, MS; Soares, CF; Demicheli, C. Novel methods for the encapsulation of meglumine antimoniate into liposomes. *Braz. J. Med. Biol. Res.,* 2000 33,841-6.

[67] Sereno, D; Cavaleyra, M; Zemzoumi, K; Masquaire, S; Ouaissi, A; Lemesre, JL. Axenically grown amastigotes of Leishmania infantum used as an in vitro model to investigate the pentavalent antimony mode of action. Antimicrob. *Agents Chemother*,1998 42, 3097–3102.

[68] Sundar, S; More, DK; Singh, MK; Singh, VP; Sharma, S; Makharia, A et al. Failure of pentavalent antimony in visceral leishmaniasis in India:

report from the center of indian epidemic. *Clin. Infect Dis.*, 2000 31, 1104-6.

[69] Jha, TK. Evaluation of diamidine compound (pentamidine isethionate) in the treatment resistant cases of kala-azar occurring in North Bihar, India. *Trans. R. Soc. Trop. Med. Hyg.*, 1983 77, 167–70.

[70] Das, VN; Ranjan, A; Sinha, AN; Verma, N; Lal, CS; Gupta, AK et al. A randomized clinical trial of low dosage combination of pentamidine and allopurinol in the treatment of antimony unresponsive cases of visceral leishmaniasis. *J. Assoc. Physicians India,* 2001 49, 609-13.

[71] Seaman, J; Pryce, D; Sondorp, H; Wilkinson, R; Bryceson, ADM. Epidemic visceral leishmaniasis in Sudan: A randomized trial of aminosidine plus sodium stibogluconate versus sodium stibogluconate alone. *J. Infect Dis.*, 1994 168, 715-20.

[72] Sundar, S; Jha, TK; Thakur, CP; Sinha, PK; Bhattacharya, SK. Injectable paromomycin for visceral leishmaniasis in India. *N. Engl. J. Med.,* 2007 356, 2571–2581.

[73] Thakur, CP; Kanyok, TP; Pandey, AK; Sinha, GP; Messick, C; Olliaro, PA. Prospective randomized, comparative, open-label trial of the safety and efficacy of paromomycin (aminosidine) plus sodium stibogluconate versus sodium stibogluconate alone for the treatment of visceral leishmaniasis. *Trans. R. Soc. Trop. Med. Hyg.*, 2000 94, 429-31.

[74] Urbina, JA. Lipid biosynthesis pathways as chemotherapeutic targets in kinetoplastid parasites. *Parasitology,* 1997 114(Suppl),S91-S9.

[75] Murray, HW; Delph-Etienne, S. Visceral leishmanicidal activity of hexadecylphosphocholine (miltefosine) in mice deficient in T cells and activated macrophage microbicidal mechanisms. *J. Infect Dis.,* 2000 181, 795-9.

[76] Sundar, S; Jha, TK; Thakur, CP; Engel, J; Sindermann, H; Fischer, C; Junge, K; Bryceson, A; Berman, J. Oral miltefosine for indian leishmanisis. *N. Engl. J. Med.*, 2002 347, 1739-46.

[77] Bhattacharya, SK; Sinha, PK; Sundar, S etal. Phase 4 trial of miltefosine for the treatment of Indian visceral leishmaniasis. *J. Infect Dis.,* 2007 196, 591–598.

[78] Gradoni L, Soteriadou K, Louzir H, Dakkak A, Toz SO, Jaffe C, Dedet JP, Campino L, Cañavate C, Dujardin JC. Drug regimens for visceral leishmaniasis in Mediterranean countries. *Trop. Med. Int. Health*. 2008 Oct;13(10):1272-6.

[79] Thakur, CP; Singh, RK; Hassan, SM; Kumar, R; Narain, S; Kumar, A. Amphotericin B deoxycholate treatment of visceral leishmaniasis with

newer modes of administration and precautions: a study of 938 cases. *Trans. R. Soc. Trop. Med. Hyg.*,1999 93, 319–323.

[80] Sundar, S; Gupta, LB; Rastogi, V; Agrawall, G; Murray, HW. Short course, cost-effective treatment with Amphotericin B-fat emulsion cures visceral leishmaniasis. *Trans. R. Soc. Trop. Med. Hyg.,* 2000 94, 200-4.

[81] Meyerhoff, A. U.S. Food and Drug Administration approval of AmBisome (liposomal amphotericin B) for treatment of visceral leishmaniasis. *Clin. Infect Dis.*, 1999 28, 42–48.

[82] Dietze, R; Fagundes, SMS; Brito, EF et al. Treatment of kalaazar in Brazil with Amphocil (amphotericin B cholesterol dispersion) for 5 days. *Trans. R. Soc. Trop. Med. Hyg.*, 1995 89, 309–311.

[83] Gaeta, GB; Maisto, A; Di Caprio, D et al. Efficacy of amphotericin B colloidal dispersion in the treatment of Mediterranean visceral leishmaniasis in immunocompetent adult patients. *Scand. J. Infect. Dis.*, 2000 32, 675–677.

[84] Sundar, S; Agrawal, NK; Sinha, PR; Horwith, GS; Murray, HW. Short-course, low dose amphotericin B lipid complex therapy for visceral leishmaniasis unresponsive to antimony. *Ann. Intern. Med.* 1997 127, 133–137.

[85] Sundar, S; Jha, TK; Thakur, CP et al. Single-dose liposomal amphotericin B in the treatment of visceral leishmaniasis in India: a multicenter study. *Clin. Infect Dis.,* 2003 37, 800–4.

[86] Syriopoulou, V; Daikos, GL; Theodoridou, M et al. Two doses of a lipid formulation of amphotericin B for the treatment of Mediterranean visceral leishmaniasis. *Clin. Infect Dis.*, 2003 36, 560–6.

[87] Sundar, S; Agrawal, G; Rai, M et al. Treatment of Indian visceral leishmaniasis with single or daily infusions of low dose liposomal amphotericin B: randomized trial. *BMJ*, 2001 323, 419–22.

[88] Murray, HW. Treatment of visceral leishmaniasis (kala-azar): a decade of progress and future approaches. *Int. J. Infect. Dis.,* 2000 4, 158-77.

[89] Sherwood, JA; Gachihi, GS; Muiggai, RK; Skillman, DR; Mugo, M; Rashid, JR et al. Phase 2 efficacy trial of an oral 8-aminoquinoline (WR6026) for treatment of visceral leishmaniasis. *Clin. Infect Dis.*, 1994 19, 1034-9.

[90] Dietze, R; Carvalho, SF; Valli, LCet al. Phase 2 trial of WR6026, an orally administered 8-aminoquinoline, in the treatment of visceral leishmaniasis caused by Leishmania chagasi. *Am. J. Trop. Med. Hyg.*, 2001 65, 685-9.

[91] Sundar, S; Murray, HW. Effect of treatment with interferon-gamma alone in visceral leishmaniasis. *J. Infect Dis.*, 1995 172, 1627-9.

[92] Badaro, R; Falcoff, E; Badaro, FS; Carvalho, EM; Pedral-Sampaio, D; Barral, A Carvalho JS, Barral-Netto M, Brandely M, Silva L, et al.Treatment of visceral leishmaniasis with pentavalent antimony and interferon gamma. *N. Engl. J. Med.*, 1990 322, 16-21.

[93] Khalil, EAG; El Hassan, AM; Zijlstra, EE et al. Autoclaved Leishmania major vaccine for prevention of visceral leishmaniasis: a randomised, double-blind, BCG-controlled trial in Sudan. *Lancet,* 2000 356, 1565–9.

In: Leishmaniasis
Editor: Carlos Sepulveda

ISBN: 978-1-62417-700-2

Chapter 3

The Role of Neutrophils in Visceral Leishmaniasis

Aline de A. Carvalho and Francisco A. L. Costa*
Departamento de Clínica e Cirurgia Veterinária,
Setor de Patologia Animal, Centro de Ciências Agrárias,
Universidade Federal do Piauí, Brazil

Abstract

Visceral Leishmaniasis (VL) is endemic in Brazil and has great economic and social impact. Each year, approximately 3,156 cases are recorded, with 10% mortality. The most important reservoir is the dog, which is an excellent model for the study of VL. VL is immune mediated, and most studies are directed toward the understanding of acquired immunity, both humoral and cellular. More recently, the role of innate immunity in VL has been the target of investigations. Neutrophils are the major leucocytic cell effectors of the innate immune response because in the course of VL, neutrophils are rapidly recruited to the site of parasite inoculation, but their role in the modulation of infection is not well defined. Neutrophils secrete lytic enzymes and nitric oxide, which cause the death of many pathogens, thus participating in the elimination of microorganisms by phagocytosis, which is mediated by opsonins, the

* Corresponding author: Francisco Assis Lima Costa, Universidade Federal do Piauí, Centro de Ciências Agrárias, Departamento de Clinica e Cirurgia Veterinária, Setor de patologia Animal, 64049-550, Campus Socopo- S/N, Teresina, Piauí, Brasil. Telephone: + 55 (86) 3215 5760, Fax number: + 55 86 3215 5753, e-mail: fassisle@gmail.com.

Toll-like receptor family, and lipopolysaccharides. The activity of neutrophils in Leishmania infection has been studied in murine models of the cutaneous form of the disease and appears to play a protective role by killing the parasites in the acute phase but not in chronic infections. In vitro experiments with human neutrophils infected with *L. donovani* demonstrate that the death of intracellular parasites is carried out by the H_2O_2-peroxidase-halide system. BALB/c mice infected with *L. donovani* and depleted of neutrophils show an increase in the number of parasites in the spleen and bone marrow and a reduction of the formation of granulomas in the liver, with a reduction in nitric oxide synthesis. The immune response against the parasite in the absence of neutrophils is altered with increased IL-10 and IL-4 in the serum and spleen and a decrease in CD4+ and CD8+ T cells producing IFN, suggesting that in the absence of neutrophils, the Th1-type immune response is compromised. Moreover, *Leishmania* may use the neutrophil as a mechanism of escape when phagocytized in non-lytic compartments that present markers of the endoplasmic reticulum and are unable to merge with lysosomal organelles. The lpg1 and lpg2 genes, which encode *Leishmania* phosphoglycans, are clearly involved in the ability of the parasite to remain in these compartments, preventing their degradation and delaying neutrophil apoptosis to increase their life span in the cells. In vitro, co-incubation of polymorphonuclear neutrophils (PMNs) with promastigotes of *L. major* leads to the inhibition of the spontaneous apoptosis of neutrophils, resulting in intracellular survival of the parasite. After infection, PMN eventually undergo apoptosis. Phosphatidyl serine is exposed on the surface of apoptotic PMN, leading to their recognition and phagocytosis by macrophages and thus contributing to the maintenance of infection. The aim of this review is to perform a critical analysis of various factors involved in the participation of neutrophils in VL.

Keywords: Visceral leishmaniasis, neutrophils, parasitology

1. Introduction

Visceral Leishmaniasis (VL) is a zoonosis that is endemic in 98 countries, with a worldwide incidence of 500,000 cases per year. Ninety percent of global VL occurs in six countries: India, Bangladesh, Sudan, South Sudan, Ethiopia and Brazil (WHO, 2012).

Unlike other endemic countries, India is the only country in which the disease can be transmitted without the participation of an animal reservoir and may be transmitted with only the involvement of a human reservoir and the sandfly vector. Currently, the epidemiology of VL has been changing drastically due to expansion into new areas, such as in Brazil (Oliveira et al., 2006), and an increased rate of co-infection with HIV, particularly in European countries (WHO, 2012).

According to the World Health Organization (WHO), 70% of HIV cases in southern Europe are also co-infected with visceral leishmaniasis. In Brazil, the disease is caused by *Leishmania* (*Leishmania*) *chagasi* (= *L.* (*Leishmania*) *infantum chagasi*) (Shaw et al., 2006) and transmitted by the bite of the female phlebotomine sandfly species *Lutzomyia longipalpis* and *Lutzomyia cruzi* (Santos et al, 1998; Monteiro et al., 2005; BRAZIL, 2006).

In endemic areas, canine visceral leishmaniasis (CVL) is considered to be more important than the human disease because infected dogs have a high parasitic load on their skin, making them the primary source of infection for the vectors (Marzochi et al., 1985).

Both the human and canine diseases are immunologically mediated, and most studies are directed toward the understanding of acquired immunity, humoral and cellular. The disease appears to develop according to the anergic model, inducing the suppression of T cells, polyclonal activation of B cells, and specific and nonspecific antibody production, culminating in the formation of high levels of anti-*Leishmania* antibodies and circulating immune complexes (Slappendel, 1988; Abranches, Santos, Gomes, 1985; Costa, 2012). Specific cellular immunity appears to be related to the cellular response that is associated with the activation of Th1 cells producing IFN-γ, IL-2, TNF-α□ and antigen-specific IgG-2 (Pinelli et al, 1994; Reis et al., 2006; Costa, 2012). Only recently has the role of innate immunity in VL been the target of investigations.

Neutrophils are major leucocytic cell effectors of the innate immune response, secreting lytic enzymes and nitric oxide that cause the death of many pathogens, including *Leishmania*. These cells have different behaviors against *Leishmania* infection. The parasites can be killed by phagocytosis even before being engulfed by the release of a Neutrophil Extracellular Trap (NETs) (Guimarães-Costa et al., 2009), or they develop evasion mechanisms with the formation of non-lytic vacuoles that present endoplasmic reticulum markers in which the parasites survive (Gueirard et al., 2008), or they can inhibit the apoptotic death of neutrophils, enhancing their survival and spread by the macrophages that phagocytose parasitized neutrophils (Aga et al., 2002).

2. Interaction of Neutrophils with Infectious Agents

In response to infection, different types of cells react, resulting in the secretion of numerous factors that trigger activation and modulation (Hurst, 2011). In humans, neutrophils are numerous leukocytes that comprise approximately 40 to 70% of peripheral blood cells under normal conditions. The average lifespan of neutrophils in the circulatory system is 6 to 10 hours, but after activation and migration into tissue, this time increases to 2 to 6 days, thus delaying death by apoptosis. Neutrophil activation occurs because of stimuli that enable cell migration to the site of injury and destruction of the pathogen, constituting a fundamental mechanism in innate immunity (Hurst, 2011). Upon reaching the injured organ, neutrophils recognize the causative agent of injury by membrane receptors, triggering phagocytosis of particles and microorganisms and their subsequent destruction by reactive oxygen species (ROS) and proteolytic proteins and antimicrobicides. After this process, neutrophils undergo apoptosis and are phagocytosed by macrophages (Theilgaard-Monch et al., 2006).

In mediating infection, neutrophils release granules that clear microorganisms through the action of enzymes that lead to the hydrolytic degradation of the substrate. The three main types of granules are the azurophilic granules or primary, secondary or specific granules and granules of gelatinase or tertiary (Borregaard and Cowland, 1997; Faurschou and Borregaard, 2003). The azurophilic granules contain antimicrobicide proteins present in granular membranes, including CD63, which are responsible for the release of granules; CD68, which induces endocytosis and lysosomal trafficking; and presenilin 1, which acts proteolytically (Holness and Simmons, 1993). The specific or secondary and tertiary or gelatinase granules are peroxidase-negative. The specific granules also act as antimicrobials after degranulation in the phagosome and extracellular medium. Some proteins that act as antimicrobial agents are the natural resistance-associated macrophage protein 1 (Nramp-1), lactoferrin, cathelicidin (HCAF-18) and lysozyme. Gelatinase granules act in the movement of neutrophils through membrane receptors that bind neutrophils after this movement. Both peroxidase-negative granules contain the p22gp91 PHOX complex (cytochrome b558), components of the NADPH oxidase complex that are responsible for the drift of electrons in the respiratory burst (Borregaard and Cowland, 1997; Faurschou and Borregaard, 2003).

In infections with *Escherichia coli* and *Staphylococcus aureus*, the neutrophil plays an important role in the killing of the microorganisms by phagocytes through the generation and release of lytic enzymes and the production of nitric oxide (Cassatella, 1999; Nathan, 2006). In the process of phagocytosis, neutrophils recognize the pathogen or injured tissue via receptors, emitting membrane extensions to cover the agent. Phagocytosis may be mediated by opsonins such as immunoglobulin G and complement fractions C3b and C3bi. There is also involvement of ligand activators of neutrophils, such as the Toll family receptors (Toll-like receptors TLR2 and TLR4), which are receptors for particles and lipopolysaccharides (Tuon et al., 2008). During the phagocytic process, neutrophils emit pseudopodia with receptors that bind the particles being phagocytosed to form vesicles (the phagosome). Along with this process, the NADPH oxidase complex is formed, which produces superoxide anions. Superoxide anions are the primary material for various oxidants such as oxidative halogens, free radicals and free oxygen in a reaction known as respiratory burst, which is very important for the destruction of the pathogen.

During bacterial infections, lipopolysaccharide (LPS) and formyl-methionyl-leucyl-phenylalanine (fMPL), present on the cell membrane of pathogens, are neutrophil activators that act as chemoattractants. When neutrophils reach the site of infection, bacteria are generally opsonized, which tells the neutrophils to perform phagocytosis. In inflammation without infection, other chemokines, such as tumor necrosis factor alpha (TNF-α), interleukins, and platelet activating factor (PAF), are released by leukocytes and tissues after tissue injury, achieving neutrophil chemotaxis with lithic granule release. In both types of inflammation (infectious or non-infectious), the balance between recruitment, the release of toxic substances and neutrophil apoptosis is critical for the inflammatory agent to be eradicated, and the response is gradually discontinued. Some diseases that are aggravated by the loss of this imbalance can present complications and multiple organ dysfunctions (Hurst, 2011).

3. The Immune Response in Visceral Leishmaniasis

VL is an immune-mediated disease, but the immunological events related to resistance and susceptibility are not well defined. Studies of VL indicate a mixed Th1 and Th2 response in that the control of parasite replication and the progression of disease or healing is determined by the balance between the two patterns (Baneth et al., 2008). However, it has been observed that dogs that are resistant to infection tend to exhibit an immune response that includes Th1-mediated CD4+ and CD8+ cells and the production of IL-2, IL-12, IFNγ, TNFα, leading to the activation of phagocytic mononuclear cells, primarily macrophages and neutrophils, which results in the production of the L-arginine and nitric oxide that are responsible for the destruction of intracellular amastigotes. Moreover, dogs susceptible to disease are characterized by severe clinical development that appears to be related to the formation of immunocomplexes resulting from a Th2 immune response with the production of IL-4, IL-5, IL-6, IL-10 and the proliferation of B lymphocytes, which are not protective (Barbieri, 2006).

IL-10 may promote an increase in the Th2 response, blocking the proliferation of Th1 cells. IL-4 induces the production of B lymphocytes, promoting a Th2-type response with an increase of serum levels of IgE and IgG1 immunoglobulins (Varella and Strong, 2001). These immunoglobulins can be strongly associated with a severe clinical picture of canine VL (Quinnell et al., 2001).

Experiments with BALB/c mice infected with *L. donovani* that used specific depletion of neutrophils showed a significant increase in the number of parasites in the spleen and bone marrow of the animals and a delay in the formation of granulomas in the liver, with decreased synthesis of nitric oxide. The immune response against the parasite in the absence of neutrophils appears to be changed, as the results show an increase in the serum and spleen of IL-10 and IL-4 and a decrease in CD4+ and CD8+ cells producing IFN, suggesting that in the absence of neutrophils, the development of a Th1-type immune response is impaired. All of these results indicate the involvement of neutrophils in resistance to infection by *L. donovani* and the subsequent development of an immune response (McFarlane et al., 2008).

Patients with VL appear to suffer from an acquired IL-8 deficiency with abnormal neutrophil activation potential (Elshafie et al., 2011), but this statement does not apply to the whole process of modulation of VL, as it has been observed that the induction of IL-8 secretion by *L. donovani* suggests a role of this cytokine in the early recruitment of neutrophils to the site of infection (Badolato et al., 1996).

Symptomatic dogs generally have high titers of anti-*Leishmania* antibodies, while those resistant to infection present with low levels or absence of antibodies (Cunt et al., 2000; Galleno-Solano et al., 2001). The immunoglobulin IgG2 appears to be associated with asymptomatic infection (Deplazes et al., 1995). Many aspects of the pathogenesis of canine VL are due

including changes in chromatin and cytoplasmatic vacuolization (Masina et al., 2007).

The action of neutrophils against *Leishmania* infection appears to depend on intrinsic factors of the host such as the host's immune status, as well as the parasite's development of adaptation mechanisms and escape from the microbicidal action of neutrophils. Neutrophils may allow "silent" entry of *Leishmania* (Chang et al., 1993; Charmoy et al., 2007). Phagocytosis of *Leishmania donovani* promastigotes by neutrophils can cause the formation of phagosomes that present markers of the endoplasmic reticulum, which do not fuse with lysosomes, allowing the survival of the parasite. Phosphoglycans and the presence of genes *lpg1* and *lpg2* are clearly involved in the ability of the parasite to persist in these compartments, thus preventing its degradation. (Gueirard et al.. 2008). Moreover, the catalytic activity of the acid phosphatase enzyme of the parasite inhibits production of superoxide anion by neutrophils when stimulated by fMPL. Acid phosphatase present in the surface of *L. donovani* can interfere with the ability of phagocytes to kill the parasite (Ramaley et al., 1984). This enzyme catalyzes the dephosphorylation of phosphoproteins, including histones, which can affect the activation of phagocytic cells that are regulated by the phosphorylation and dephosphorylation of membrane proteins (Andrews and Babior, 1983; Huang et al., 1984). The capacity of survival of *Leishmania* within neutrophils is also related to the inhibition of the fusion of phagosomes that contain *Leishmania* by secondary and tertiary granules, which inactivates the respiratory burst (Mollinedo et al., 2010). Only fusion of azurophilic granules with leishmania-containing phagosomes can release arginase I from these granules, which facilitates the survival of the parasite (Iniesta, Gomez-Nieto, Corraliza, 2001; Munder et al., 2005).

The mechanism of suppression of neutrophil apoptosis by phagocytosed *Leishmania* appears to be another escape mechanism of the parasite. A co-incubation experiment of polymorphonuclear (PMN) with promastigotes of *L. major* in vitro led to the inhibition of spontaneous apoptosis of the neutrophils, resulting in intracellular survival of the parasite. After infection, the PMN eventually underwent apoptosis. Phosphatidyl serine, when exposed on the surface of apoptotic PMN, leads to their recognition and phagocytosis by macrophages and thus contributes to the maintenance and dissemination of infection (Scianimanico et al., 1999; Dermine et al., 2000; Aga et al., 2002; Gueirard et al., 2008) because infected neutrophils and monocytes attract macrophages to the site of infection by producing a chemotactic protein known as MIP-1 (Wang et al., 1993). The inhibition of neutrophil apoptosis by

Leishmania is associated with a decrease in the activity of caspase-3, which suggests that *L. major* affects the transformation of procaspase-3 to enzymatically active caspase-3. Therefore, the transition of procaspase-3 to caspase-3 appears to be an action performed by *L. major* to inhibit the spontaneous apoptosis of PMN (Aga et al.. 2002).

In VL, the involvement of the CXCR1 or CXCR2 receptors appears to play a role in the chemotaxis and activation of the PMN to the site of infection (Stillie et al., 2009). Both receptors have high affinity for the CXC chemokines of IL-8, as CXCR1 is specific for IL-8 (Peters et al., 2008; McFarlane et al., 2008). Elevated levels of CXCL8 are present in dogs with high cutaneous parasitism, which induces chemotaxis and neutrophil influx to the infected tissue, contributing to parasite survival (Van Zandbergen et al., 2004). Interestingly, it has been reported that the parasite produces a protein with chemotactic properties, called factor chemotactic for leishmania, which promotes the migration of neutrophils to the site of infection (Van Zandbergen et al., 2002), causing the phagocytosis of these parasites. A study evaluating the initial events that occur in the skin during infection by *Leishmania major* revealed that the decrease of neutrophils in these animals was associated with an inability of the parasite to establish infection (Peters et al., 2008). Furthermore, a mixed cytokine profile has been observed in VL, with a predominance of cutaneous levels of IL-10 and TGF-β1 and with less expression of IL-12, which may be a prerequisite for the persistence of the parasite and replication in the skin (Menezes-Souza et al., 2011).

5. Final Considerations

The role of neutrophils in visceral leishmaniasis is complex and requires further study. Visceral leishmaniasis is an immunologically mediated disease with a strong contribution from the acquired immune system, humoral and cellular, where the organic alterations vary from individual to individual and from organ to organ, depending on the degree of parasitization and the response of the host against infection. Neutrophils, as innate immunity cells, both act in the control of infection in well-defined phases and are controlled by it when the parasite develops adaptive mechanisms and escapes. This dichotomy appears to be due to the balance of the immune response in which the secretion of cytokines, antibodies and T cells plays an important role. It is likely that the initial action of neutrophils in protection against infection is replaced later by an adaptive response of the parasite to use the PMN for their survival, as occurs with the cellular host of *Leishmania major*, the macrophage. We have observed that in chronic infection with visceral leishmaniasis in naturally infected dogs, when few or no *Leishmania* amastigotes were present in the skin, the inflammatory infiltrate was composed primarily of lymphocytes and macrophages, but when many parasites were present, the infiltrate also contained lymphocytes and macrophages, as well as a larger quantity of PMNs (Verçosa et al., 2008). In dogs naturally infected with *Leishmania (L.) chagasi* that presented with clinical manifestations, we found a significant positive correlation between parasite load and the presence of neutrophils in the ear (Carvalho, 2011), suggesting that unlike in the acute infection, in chronic infection, neutrophils contribute to the survival of the parasite, either by inhibiting the formation of lytic phagosomes, by inhibiting neutrophil death by apoptosis, or by the increased secretion of chemokines, which determine the flow of neutrophils to the site of injury. Thus, we believe that neutrophils constitute an important cell in the pathogenesis of *Leishmania* infection whose action contributes to the understanding of the mechanism of interaction of the parasite with the host.

References

Abranches, P.; Santos, C. L; Gomes, G. M., 1998. "Canine Leishmaniasis: New Concepts in Epidemiology and Im-munology and Their Reflections in the Control of Human Visceral Leishmaniasis," *Acta Médica Portuguesa*. 11, 871-875.

Agar. E., Katschinski, D. M., Zandbergen, G. V.; Laufs, H., Hansen, B., Muller, K., Solbach, w., Laskay, T., 2002. Inhibition of the spontaneous apoptosis of neutrophil granulocytes by the intracellular parasite Leishmania major. *The Journal of Immunology*. 169, 898-905.

Andrews, P. C., and Babior, B. M., 1983. Endogenous protein phosphorylation by resting and activated human neutrophils *Blood* 61, 333-340.

Badatolo, R.; Sacks, D. L.; Savoia, D.; Musso, T., 1996. Leishmania Major: infection of human monocytes induces expression of IL-8 and MCAF. *Exp. Parasitol.* 82, 21-26.

Baneth, G.; Koutinas, A. F.; Solano-Gallego, L.; Bourdeau, P.; Ferrer, L., 2008. "Canine leishmaniosis - new concepts and insights on an expanding zoonosis: part one", *Trends in Parasitology*. 24, 324-330.

Barbieri, C. L., 2006. Immunology of canine leishmaniasis. *Parasite Immunology*.28, 329-337.

Berger, M., J. O'Shea, A. S. Cross, T. M. Folks, T. M. Chused, E. J. Brown,and M. M. Frank**.,** 1984. Human neutrophils increase expression of C3bi as well as C3b receptors upon activation. *J. Clin. Investig.* 74,1566–1571.

Boceta, C.; Alonso, C.; Jimenez-Ruiz, A., 2000. Leucine rich repeats are the main epitopes in Leishmania infantum PSA during canine and human visceral leishmaniasis. *Parasite Immunology*.22, 55-62.

Borregaard, N.; Cowland, J. B., 1997. Granules of the human neutrophil polymorphonuclear leukocyte. *Blood*, 89, 3502-3521.

BRASIL-Ministério da Saúde., 2006. Secretaria de Vigilância em Saúde. Departamento de Vigilância Epidemiológica. *Manual de Vigilância e Controle da Leishmaniose Visceral. Brasília: Editora do ministério da Saúde.*

Carvalho, A. A. Diagnóstico parasitológico de leishmaniose visceral canina e sua associação com o infiltrado inflamatório neutrofílico. 2011.57f. Dissertação (mestrado em ciência animal) *Centro de Ciência Agrária.* Universidade Federal do Piauí. Teresina. Piauí, 2011

Cassatella, M. A., 1999. Neutrophil-derived proteins: selling cytokines by the pound. *Advances in immunology*.73, 369.

Chang, H. R.; Vesin, C.; Grau, G. E.; Pointaire, P.; Arsenijevic, D.; Strath, M.; Pechere, J. C.; Piguet, P. F., 1993. Respective role of polymorphonuclear leukocytes and their integrins (CD-11/18) in the local or systemic toxicity of[lipopolysaccharide. *Journal of leukocyte biology*.53, 636–639.

Charmoy, M.; Megnekou, R.; Allenbach, C; Zweifel, C.; Perez, C.; Monnat, K.; Breton, M.; Ronet, C.; Launois, P.;Tacchini-Cottier, F., 2007. *Leishmania major* induces distinct neutrophil phenotypes in mice that are resistant or susceptible to infection. *Journal of leukocyte biology*. 82, 288–299.

Chen, L., Zhang, Z. H.; Watanabe, T.; Yamashita, T.; Kobayakawa, T.; Kaneko, A.; Fujiwara, H.; Sendo. F., 2005. The involvement of neutrophils in the resistance to *Leishmania major* infection in susceptible but not in resistant mice. *Parasitology international*. 54, 109–118..

Costa, F.A.L., 2012. The dog as a risck factor in transmission of visceral leishmaniasis: A review. *Advances in infectious disease*..2, 37-47.

Dermine, J.F., Scianimanico, S., Prive, C., Descoteaux, A.; Desjardins, M., 2000. *Leishmania* promastigotesrequire lipophosphoglycan to actively modulate the fusionproperties of phagosomes at an early step of phagocytosis. *Cell Microbiol.* 2, 115–126.

Elshafie, A. I.; Ahlin, E.; Hakonsson, L. D.; Elghazali, G.; Safi, S. H.; Ronnelid, J.; Venge, P., 2011. Activity and turnover of eosinophil and neutrophil granulocytes are altered in visceral leishmaniasis. *International Journal for Parasitology*.41,463-469.

Engwerda, C. R.; Smelt, S. C. ; Kaye, P. M., 1996. An in vivo analysis of cytokine production during Leishmania donovani infection in scid mice. *Exp. Parasitol.*84,195-201.

Faurschou, M.; Borregaard, N., 2003. Neutrophil granules and secretoty vesicles in inflammation. *Microbes Infect*, 5, 1317-1327.

Fuchs T. A,; Abed, U.; Goosmann, C.; Hurwitz, R.; Schulze, I.; Wahn, V.; Weinrauch, Y.; Brinkmann, V., 2007. Novel cell death program leads to neutrophil extracellular traps. *J Cell Biol*. 176, 231–241.

Gueirard P, Laplante A, Rondeau C, Milon G, Desjardins M., 2008. Trafficking of *Leishmania donovani* promastigotes in nonlytic compartments in neutrophils enables the subsequent transfer of parasites to macrophages. *Cell Microbiol.* 10, 100–111.

Guimaraes-Costa A. B, Nascimento M. T, Froment G. S, Soares R. P, Morgado F. N, Conceicao-Silva F, Saraiva E.M., 2009. Leishmania amazonensis promastigotes induce and are killed by neutrophil extracellular traps. *Proc Natl Acad Sci U S A*.16,6748-6753.

Holness, C. L.; Simnons, D. L., 1993. Molecular cloning of CD68, a human macrophage marker related to lyssomal glycoproteins. *Blood*, 81, 1607 - 1617.

Huang, C. K., Oshana, S. C., and Becker, E. L, 1984. A phosphoprotein of 90,000 Mr. that copurifies with the formylpeptide receptor of rabbit peritoneal neutrophils, *Fed. Proc.* 43,1417.

Hurst, J. K., 2012. What really happens in the neutrophil phagosome? *Free Radical Biology and Medicine*. 53, 508-520.

Iniesta, V.; Gomez-Nieto, L. C.; Corraliza, I., 2001. The Inhibition of Arginase by N^{ω}-Hydroxy-L-Arginine Controls the Growth of *Leishmania* Inside Macrophages. *J. Exp. Med.* 193, 777–784.

Laufs, H., Muller, K., Fleischer, J., Reiling, N., Jahnker, N., Jensenius, J. C., Salbach, W., Laskay, T., 2002. Intracellular survival of Leishmania major in neutrophil granulocytes after uptake in the absence of heat-labile serum factors. *Infection and Immunity*.70, .826-835.

Lima, G. M.; Vallochi, A. L.; Silva, U. R.; Bevilacqua, E. M.; Kiffer, M. M.; Abrahamsohn, I. A., 1998. The role of polymorphonuclear leukocytes in the resistance to cutaneous Leishmaniasis. *Immunology letters*. 64, 145–151.

Marzochi, M. C. A. ; Coutinho, S. G.; Sabroza, P. C. ; Souz, M. A.; Souza, P. P. ; Toledo, L. M.; Rangel Filho, F. B., 1985. "Leishmaniose Visceral Canina no Rio de Janeiro Brasil," *Cadernos de Saúde Pública*. 1, 432-446.

Masina S.; Zangger H.; Rivier D.; Fasel, N., 2007. Histone H1 regulates chromatin condensation in *Leishmania* parasites. *Exp Parasitol.* 116, 83–87.

McFarlane E, Perez C, Charmoy M, Allenbach C, Carter K. C, Alexander J, Tacchini-Cottier F., 2008. Neutrophils contribute to development of a protective immune response during onset of infection with *Leishmania donovani*. *Infect Immun*. 76,532-541.

Menezes-Souza D, Correa-Oliveira R, Guerra-Sa R, Giunchetti RC, Teixeira-Carvalho A, Martins-Filho, O. A.; Oliveira, G. C.; Reis, A. B., 2011. Cytokine and transcription factor profiles in the skin of dogs naturally infected by Leishmania (Leishmania) chagasi presenting distinct cutaneous parasite density and clinical status. *Vet Parasitol*. 177, 39–49.

Mollinedo, F.; Janssen. H.; Iglesia-Vicente, J.; Villa-Pulgarin, J. A.; Calafat, J., 2010. Selective Fusion of Azurophilic Granules with *Leishmania* containing Phagosomes in Human Neutrophils, *the journal of biological chemis*try.. 285, 34528–34536.

Monteiro, E. M.; Silva, J. F. C.; Costa, R. T.; Costa, D. C.; Barata, R. A.; Paula, E. V.; Machado-Coelho, G. L. L.; Fortes-Dias, C. L.; Dias, E. S., 2005. Leishmaniose visceral: estudo de flebótomos e infecção canina em Montes Claros, Minas Gerais. *Revista da Sociedade de Medicina Tropical*.1, 147-157.

Mosser, D. M., H. Vlassara, P. J. Edelson, and A. Cerami., 1987. Leishmania promastigotes are recognized by the macrophage receptor for advanced glycosylation endproducts. *J. Exp. Med*. 165, 140–145.

Munder, M., Mollinedo, F., Calafat, J., Canchado, J., Gil-Lamaignere, C.,Fuentes, J. M., Luckner, C., Doschko, G., Soler, G., Eichmann, K., Mu¨ller,F. M., Ho, A. D., Goerner, M., and Modolell, M., 2005. Arginase I is constitutively expressed in human granulocytes and participates in fungicidal activity. *Blood*. 105, 2549–2556.

Murray, H. W. and Nathan, C. F., 1999. macrophage microbicidal mechanisms in vivo: reactive nitrogen versus oxygens intermediates in the killing of intracellular visceral Leishmania donovani. *J. Exp. Med*.189,.741-747.

Nathan, C., 2006. Neutrophils and immunity: challenges and opportunities. Nature reviews. *Immunology*. 6, 173–182.

Oliveira, A. L. L.; Paniago, A. M. M.; Dorval, M. E. L.; Oshiro, E. T.; Leal, C. R.; Sanches, M.; Cunha, R. V.; Boia, M. N., 2006. Foco Emergente de leishmaniose Visceral em Mato Grosso do Sul. *Revista da Sociedade Brasileira de medicina Tropical.*39,446-450.

Pearson, R. D.; Steigbigel, R. T., 1981. Phagocytosis and killing of the protozoan Leishmania donovani by human polymorphonuclear leukocytes. *The Journal of immunology.*127, 1438–1443.

Peters N. C, Egen J. G, Secundino N, Debrabant A, Kimblin N, Kamhawi S, Lawyer P, Fay M. P,Germain R. N, Sacks D., 2008. In vivo imaging reveals an essential role for neutrophils inleishmaniasis transmitted by sand flies. *Science*. 321,970-974.

Pinelli, E.; Killick-Kendrick, R.; Wagenaar, J.; Bernadina, W.; del Real, G.; Ruitenberg, J., 1994."Cellular and Humoral Im-mune Responses in *Dogs* Experimentally and Naturally Infected with *Leishmania infantum*," *Infection and Im-munity*. 62, 229-235.

Puentes, S. M., D. L. Sacks, R. P. da Silva, and K. A. Joiner., 1988. Complement binding by two developmental stages of *Leishmania major* promastigotas varying in expression of a surface lipophosphoglycan. *J. Exp. Med.* 167, 887–902.

Quinnell, R. J. Courtnay, O.; Shaw. M.; Day, M. J.; Garcez, L. M.; Dye, C.; Kaye, P. M.,2001. Tissue cytocine responses in canine visceral leishmaniasis. *Journal of Infectious Diseasis.*183, 1421-1424.

Reis, A. B.; Teixeira-Carvalho, A.; Vale, A. M; Marques, M. J. ; Giunchetti, R. C. ; Mayrink, W.; Guerra, L. L.; Andrade, R. A.; Corrêa-Oliveira, R.; Martins-Filho, O. A., 2006. "Isotype Patterns of Immunoglobulins: Hallmarks for Clinical Status and Tissue Parasite Density in Brazilian Dogs Naturally Infected by *Leishmania* (*Leishmania*) *chagasi*," *Veterinary Immunology and Immunopathology.*112, 102-116.

Remaley, A.T., Kuhns, D.B., Basford, R.E., Glew, R.H.; Kaplan, S.S., 1984. Leishmanial phosphatase blocks neutrophil O-2 production. *J* Biol Chem. 259, 11173–11175.

Ribeiro-Gomes, F. L.; Otero, A. C.; Gomes, N. A.; Moniz-de-Souza, M. C.; Rose, K.; Curtis, J.; Baldwin, T.; Mathis, A.; Kumar, B.; Sakathianadeswaren, A.; Spurck, T,; Low Choy, J.; Handman, E., 2004. Cutanius leishmaniasis in red kangaroos isolation and characterization of the causative organism. *International Journal for parasitology.*34, 655-664.

Santos, L.R., Barrouin-Melo, S.M., Chang, Y.; Olsen, J.; Mcdonough, S.P.; Quimby, F., 2004. Recombinant single-chain canine interleukin 12 induces interferon gamma mRNA expression in peripheral blood mononuclear cells of dogs with visceral leishmaniasis. *Veterinary immunology and immunopathology*. 98, 43-48.

Santos, S. O.; Arias, J.; Ribeiro, A. R.; Hoffmann, M. P.; Freitas, R. A.; Mallaco, M. A. F.,1998. Incrimination of Lutzomyia cruzi as a vector of American Visceral Leishmaniasis. *Medical and Veterinary Entomololy*.12, .315-317.

Scianimanico, S., Desrosiers, M., Dermine, J.F., Meresse, S.,Descoteaux, A., Desjardins, M.,1999. Impaired recruitment of the small GTPase rab7 correlates with the inhibition of phagosome maturation by *Leishmania donovani* promastigotes. *Cell Microbiol*. 1, 19–32.

Shaw, J.J., 2006. Further thoughts on the use of the name *Leishmania (Leishmania) infantum chagasi* for the aetiological agente of American visceral leishmaniasis. *Mem Inst Oswaldo Cruz*. 101, 577-579.

Silva-Filho F. C, Saraiva, E. M, Vannier-Santos, M. A Souza, W., 1990. The surface free energy of *Leishmania amazonensis*. Cell Biophys. 17,137–151.

Slappendel, R. J., 1988. "Canine Leishmaniasis. A Review based on 95 Cases in The Netherlands," *The Veterinary Quar-terly*. 10, 1-16.

Smett. S. C.; Cotterell, S.E.; Engwerda C. R.; Kaye, P. M., 2000. B cell-deficient mice are highly resistant to *Leishmania donovani* infection, but develop neutrophil- mediated tissue pathology. *J. Immunol*.164, 3681-3688.

Solano-Galeno, L.; Rieira, C.; Roura, X.; Iniesra, L.; Gallego, M.; Valladares, J. E.; Fisa, R.; Castillejo, S.; Alberola, J.; Ferrer, L. Arboix, M.; Portus, M., 2001. leishmaniasis infantum-specific IgG, IgG1 and IgG2 antibody response in healthy and ill dogs from endemic áreas. Evolution in the course of infection and after treatment. *Veterinary Parasitology*. 96, 265-276.

Stillie R, Farooq S. M, Gordon J. R, Stadnyk A. W., 2009. The functional significance behind expressing two IL-8 receptor types on PMN. *J Leukoc Biol*. 3, 529-543.

Thalhofer, C. J.; Chen, Y.; Sudan, B.; Love-Homan, L.; Wilso, M. E., 2011. Leukocytes infiltrate the skin and draining lymph nodes in response to the protozoan *Leishmania infantum chagasi*. *Infection and Immunity*. 79, 108-117.

Theilgaard- Mench, K.; Porse, B. T.; Borregaard, N., 2006. Systens biology of neutrophil differentiation and immune response. *Cuer. Opin Immunol.*18, 54-60.

Tuon F. F.; Amato, V. S.; Bacha, H. A.; AlMusawi, T.; Duarte, M. I.; Neto, V. A., 2008. Toll-like receptors and leishmaniasis. *Infect Immun.* 76, 866–872.

Turco S. J, Spa¨ th G. F, Beverley S. M., 2001. Is lipophosphoglycan a virulence factor? A surprising diversity between *Leishmania* species. *Trends Parasitol.* 17, 223–226.

van Zandbergen G, Hermann N, Laufs H, Solbach W, Laskay T., 2002. Leishmania promastigotes release a granulocyte chemotactic factor and induce interleukin-8 release but inhibit gamma interferon-inducible protein 10 production by neutrophil granulocytes. *Infect Immun.* 70, 4177–4184.

Varella, P. P. V.; Forte, W. C. N., 2001. Citocinas: revisão. *Revista Brasileira de Alergia e Immunopatologia.*24, 146-154.

Verçosa, B. L. A; Lemos, C. M; Mendonça, I. L; Silva, S. M. M. S; Carvalho, S. M; Goto, H; Costa, F.A.L., 2008. Transmission potencial, skin inflemmatory response and parasitismo f symptomatic and asymptomatic dogs with visceral leishmaniasis. *BMC veterinary.* 4, 45-52

Volker Brinkmann, V.; Reichard, U.; Goosmann, C.; Fauler, B.; Uhlemann, Y.; Weiss, D. S.; Weinrauch, Y.; Zychlinsky, A.,2004. Neutrophil extracellular traps kill bacteria. *Science.* 303,1532–1535.

Wang, J. M.; Sherry, B; . Fivash, M. J; . Kelvin, D. J; Oppenheim, J. J., 1993. Human recombinant macrophage inflammatory protein-1 _ and -_ and monocyte chemotactic and activating factor utilize common and unique receptors on human monocytes. *J. Immunol.* 150, 3022.

Witko-Sarsat, V., P. Rieu, B. Descamps-Latscha, P. Lesavre, and L. Halbwachs-Mecarelli., 2000. Neutrophils: molecules, functions and pathophysiological aspects. *Lab. Investig.* 80, 617–653.

World Health Organization (WHO). Contém informações institucionais, técnicas, notícias, projetos, publicações e serviços. Disponível em: *<http://www.who.int/leishmaniasis/en_>*. Acesso em 28 de Agosto de 2012.

Zandbergen G. V.; Klinger, M.; Mueller, A.; Dannenberg, S.; Gebert, A.; Solbach, W.; Laskay, T., 2004. Cutting Edger: Neutrophil granulocyte serves as a vector for Leishmania entry in macrophages. *The Journal of Immunology.*173,.6521-6525.

In: Leishmaniasis
Editor: Carlos Sepulveda

ISBN: 978-1-62417-700-2

Chapter 4

ATYPICAL MANIFESTATIONS OF CANINE VISCERAL LEISHMANIASIS

***Andréia P. Turchetti*[1], *Tatiane A. Paixão*[2] and *Renato L. Santos*[1*]**

[1] Universidade Federal de Minas Gerais, Escola de Veterinária, Dept. Clínica e Cirurgia Veterinárias. Belo Horizonte, MG, Brazil

[2] Universidade Federal de Minas Gerais, Instituto de Ciências Biológicas, Dept. Patologia Geral. Belo Horizonte, MG, Brazil

ABSTRACT

Leishmaniasis is an important zoonosis worldwide. The domestic dog is the most important reservoir in urban areas. Dogs with symptomatic visceral leishmaniasis usually present weight loss, anemia, lymphadenopathy, splenomegaly, hepatomegaly, glomerulopathy, cutaneous lesions, and onychogryphosis. However, atypical manifestations of visceral leishmaniasis have been reported, especially in endemic regions. Ocular changes such as blepharitis, keratoconjunctivitis, and anterior uveitis occur very often, but less commonly, cyclitis, chorioretinitis, retinal detachment, keratoconjunctivitis sicca associated with lacrimal gland lesions, cataract, glaucoma, and orbital cellulitis are also observed in some cases. *Leishmania* spp. has been associated with inflammatory mononuclear infiltrate in the hearth causing myocarditis, in

[*] Email: rsantos@vet.ufmg.br.

ocular-associated smooth and striated muscles, and in skeletal muscles, causing myositis. Affecting the respiratory system, sneezing with epistaxis was reported, as well as interstitial pneumonia. In the gastrointestinal tract, multiple lesions of the tongue and colitis have been reported. Polyarthritis and osteolytic osteomyelitis have been associated with leishmaniasis affecting the locomotor system. A comprehensive study of lesions in the genital system of male dogs demonstrated a very high frequency of lesions particularly in the epididymis, glans penis, and prepuce. Furthermore, dogs shed *Leishmania* spp. in the semen. Studies in bitches, however, demonstrated that vulvar dermatitis was the only important finding in the female genital system. It is known that dogs with leishmaniasis may present neurological signs. Brain inflammatory mononuclear infiltrate has been described associated with high titers of anti-*Leishmania* antibodies in the cerebrospinal fluid. There are also reports of *Leishmania* spp. causing meningitis and choroiditis. Although cutaneous lesions are often present in dogs with visceral leishmaniasis, unusual manifestations include nodular disease, sterile pustular dermatitis, discoloration of the external nares and nodular dermatofibrosis. The protozoan has been observed associated with canine transmissible venereal tumor. Amastigotes have also been found in a large numbers at other tissues in the absence of lesions. This chapter aims to describe unusual clinical signs and lesions of canine visceral leishmaniasis, and alert clinicians about the importance of including leishmaniasis in the differential diagnosis of atypical manifestations, especially in endemic regions for the disease.

INTRODUCTION

In the Americas, visceral leishmaniasis is caused by the protozoon *Leishmania (Leishmania) infantum* (synonym *L. chagasi*) and transmitted by the bite of *Lutzomyia longipalpis* sandfly. It is an important emerging zoonosis that has the domestic dog as its principal vertebrate host. *Leishmania* infects mainly cells belonging to the mononuclear phagocytic system, such as macrophages, causing chronic inflammatory processes. Therefore, clinical signs are usually related to organs that have a great number of these cells, such as bone marrow, lymph nodes, spleen and liver, causing anemia, lymphadenomegaly, splenomegaly and hepatomegaly respectively. Other common signs and lesions are weight loss, glomerulopathy by deposition of immune complex, cutaneous lesions, and onychogryphosis (reviewed by Baneth et al., 2008).

Classic canine visceral leishmaniasis appears clinically as a chronic wasting disease. However, especially in endemic regions for the disease, atypical manifestations are found. This chapter aims to describe unusual clinical signs and lesions of canine visceral leishmaniasis. It is worth saying that amastigote forms of the protozoan have been found in a large number of tissues, however, without causing lesions and, therefore, will not be discussed in this review.

Ocular Signs and Lesions

Ocular disease can be observed in approximately 25% of dogs with leishmaniasis, however, lesions restricted to the eye are rare. Ocular changes such as blepharitis, keratoconjunctivitis, and anterior uveitis occur very often in visceral leishmaniasis, but less commonly, cyclitis, chorioretinitis, retinal detachment, keratoconjunctivitis sicca associated with lacrimal gland lesions, cataract, glaucoma, and orbital cellulitis are also observed in some cases (Peña et al., 2000). We have previously reported a case of intense chronic diffuse bilateral panophthalmitis with myriad of intramacrophagic amastigotes (Figure 1) in a senile dog with visceral leishmaniasis (Carvalho Neta et al., 2007).

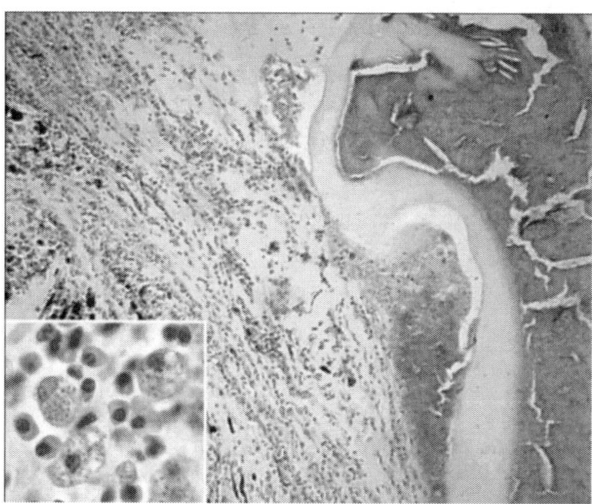

Figure 1. Panophthalmitis in a dog with visceral leishmaniasis. 18-year-old Poodle bitch with intense diffuse inflammatory infiltrate affecting iris. HE, 40x. In detail, numerous intracytoplasmic amastigotes within macrophages. HE, 1000x.

Specific anti-*Leishmania* immunoglobulin G (IgG) in the aqueous humour was confirmed in two naturally infected dogs (García-Alonso et al., 1996a). A histopathological study of the eyes demonstrated lesions affecting several ocular structures. The ciliary processes, ciliary body, sclerocorneal limbus, iris and lacrimal duct had intense inflammatory areas with mononuclear infiltrates and macrophages containing intracellular amastigote forms of *Leishmania*. In addition, vasculitis with dilation and thrombi were also detected in both cases with anti-*Leishmania* IgG. In a study including the eyes of 60 infected dogs, granulomatous inflammation was observed in 30% of the cases and *Leishmania* amastigotes in 26.6%. The most affected tissues were conjunctiva, limbus, ciliary body, iris, cornea, sclera and iridocorneal angle, choroid and the optic nerve sheath (Peña et al., 2008).

Naranjo et al. (2005) studied the atypical manifestation of keratoconjunctivitis sicca in dogs with leishmaniasis and found that their lacrimal gland ducts were surrounded by a granulomatous inflammatory infiltrate, what may produce retrograde accumulation and retention of secretion.

Leishmania was associated with granulomatous inflammation in intraocular, extraocular and adnexal smooth and striated muscles of infected dogs (Naranjo et al., 2010). Lesions and number of amastigotes were higher in striated muscles. The authors supposed that the inflammation processes could contribute to clinical signs already described, such as blepharitis, uveitis, and orbital cellulitis.

CARDIOVASCULAR SIGNS AND LESIONS

Clinical signs and lesions have been described affecting cardiovascular system of dogs with visceral leishmaniasis. Alterations in cardiac rhythm, necrotizing polyarteritis, granulomas, and non-suppurative myocarditis have been reported (Blavier et al., 2001, Torrent et al., 2005, López-Peña et al., 2009, Alves et al., 2010).

Torrent et al. (2005) reported an interesting case of myocarditis and generalized vasculitis associated with leishmaniasis. At necropsy, the epicardium showed hemorrhagic and pale areas. The last ones histologically corresponded to severe mononuclear infiltrates. There was a marking multifocal non-suppurative myocarditis of the right atrium. Vasculitis in the skin, eyes, hearth, liver, spleen and kidneys was presented and these tissues were PCR positive for *Leishmania*. Amastigotes were also seen by immunohistochemistry in the ocular tissue and in the spleen. Vasculitis was associated with a hypersensitivity reaction. Although interesting, this was not the first case of necrotizing systemic vasculitis resulting in diffuse hemorrhage in multiple organs of infected dogs (Pumarola et al., 1991).

López-Peña et al. (2009) reported a case of leishmaniasis that was seen at necropsy as large areas of pallor in the myocardium. Histological examination revealed an intense chronic inflammation in various organs, especially in the heart, where large areas of the myocardium were affected with intense mononuclear infiltrate associated to cardiac muscle atrophy and degeneration. Despite a severe inflammation, the number of parasitized macrophages tends to be low in the myocardium, as demonstrated by immunohistochemical staining of *Leishmania* amastigotes.

In a more comprehensive study, Alves et al. (2010) observed perivascular and intermuscular mononuclear inflammatory infiltrates of mild to moderate intensity in the hearth of both symptomatic and asymptomatic dogs. The protozoan was detected free in the cut on a few cases by tissue imprint and by immunohistochemistry.

Respiratory Signs and Lesions

Respiratory changes in dogs with leishmaniasis include sneezing, dyspnea, rhinitis, muco catarrhal nasal discharge, epistaxis, stertorous breath sounds, and chronic interstitial pneumonia (Slappendel, 1988, Gonçalves et al., 2003, Torrent et al., 2005, Alves et al., 2010).

Shaw et al. (2008) reported a respiratory manifestation in a dog with leishmaniasis, which had an eight-week history of intermittent sneezing and one episode of epistaxis. No nasal abnormalities were detected by radiography of the nasal cavities and there was no evidence of a foreign body. Fungal and bacterial infections as well as angiostrongyliasis were excluded and, therefore, the clinical signs were considered to be due to leishmaniasis.

The major respiratory change observed in symptomatic and asymptomatic dogs with leishmaniasis is thickening of the pulmonary alveolar septa due to mononuclear inflammation, fibrosis and congestion. Several investigators have described these well-known changes (reviewed by Gonçalves et al., 2003). However, the mechanism by which visceral leishmaniasis results in pulmonary changes is poorly understood. Alves et al. (2010) observed that in the lungs of infected dogs there was thickening of the alveolar septa due to congestion, edema, inflammatory infiltrate, and fibroblast proliferation. The protozoan was detected free or inside mononuclear cytoplasm on a few cases by tissue imprint and by immunohistochemistry. Gonçalves et al. (2003) evaluated the lungs of dogs naturally infected and found chronic and diffuse interstitial pneumonia. However, no *Leishmania* amastigote was observed in the hematoxylin and eosin staining.

Digestive Signs and Lesions

In the digestive system, atypical manifestations include mainly tongue lesions, such as nodules and glossitis or stomatitis (Figure 2), and diarrhea that is usually secondary to colitis (Ferrer et al., 1991, Blavier et al., 2001, Foglia Manzillo et al., 2005, Parpaglia et al., 2007, Viegas et al., 2012).

Non nodular ulcerative glossitis was the first report of lesions in tongue as a possible clinical sign of visceral leishmaniasis in dogs (Bourdoiseau, 2002, Lamothe & Poujade, 2002). Multiple nodular lesions of the tongue caused by *L. infantum* were reported in a symptomatic dog with the entire tongue and especially the edges taken by multiple, non-ulcerated, dome-shaped, variable in size (1–5 mm of diameter) fibrous nodules with intralesional *Leishmania* (Parpaglia et al., 2007).

Since then, two other similar cases were reported (Foglia Manzillo et al., 2009, Viegas et al., 2012). All lesions reported above regressed after appropriate treatment. An interesting case was reported by Foglia Manzillo et al. (2005), in which a dog treated for visceral leishmaniasis developed papular-like glossitis several months later. In this later case, the authors could not conclude if it was a case of reactivation and dissemination of the previous infection or a new infection with the development of localized mucosal leishmaniasis.

Ferrer et al. (1991) reported two cases of leishmaniasis in which the primary clinical sign was chronic large bowel diarrhea cursing with mucus and blood in the feces, increased frequency of defecation and low-volume stool with tenesmus and dyschezia.

A diffusely hyperemic colonic mucosa with a few focal erosions was observed upon endoscopic assessment. Biopsy of these regions revealed severe inflammatory infiltrate mainly composed by macrophages in the intestinal mucosa, muscularis mucosae and submucosa (Figure 3). In some areas, erosions characterized by the adherence of cellular debris to the surface were seen. *Leishmania* was suspected in the hematoxylin and eosin stain and confirmed by immunohistochemistry.

Other studies had already shown colitis as a possible clinical sign of leishmaniasis, however, never as the primary disease (Blavier et al., 2001). *L. infantum* may therefore be added to the list of infectious or parasitic agents causing chronic colitis such as *Salmonella* spp., *Giardia* spp. *and Balantidium* spp.

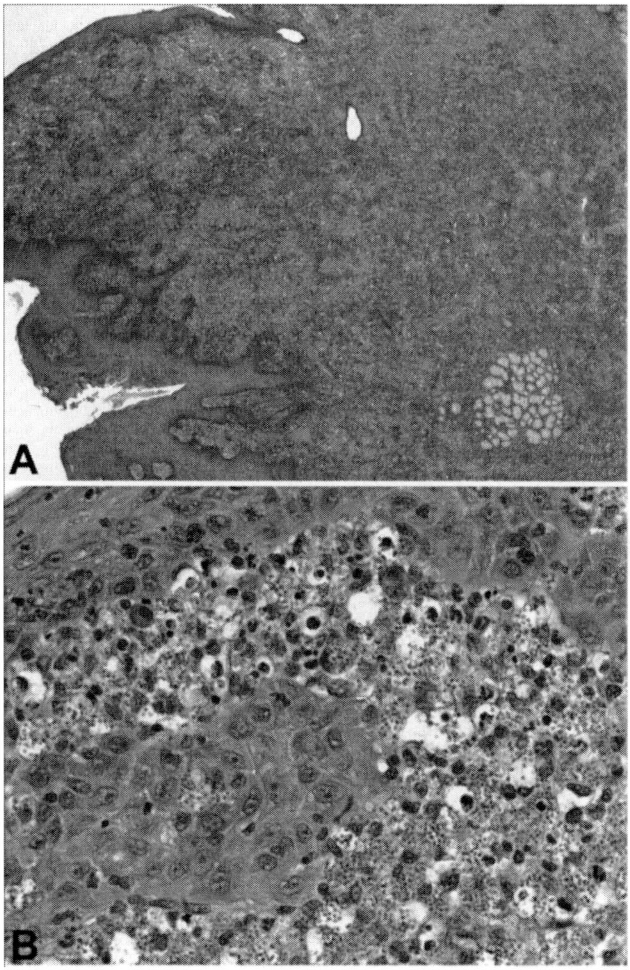

Figure 2. Stomatitis in a dog with visceral leishmaniasis. 3-year-old male Poodle with (A) a nodular lesion at the base of the tongue. HE, 40x.; with (B) intense diffuse predominantly histiocytic infiltrate with numerous intracytoplasmic amastigotes. HE, 600x.

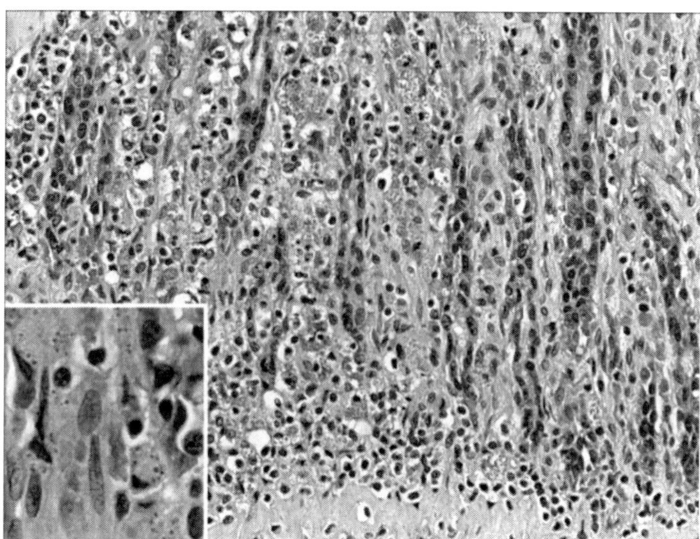

Figure 3. Enteritis in a dog with visceral leishmaniasis. 7-month-old male Fila Brasileiro with mild multifocal lympho-histio-plasmacytic infiltrate in mucosae. HE, 400x. In detail, numerous intracytoplasmic amastigotes within macrophages. HE, 1000x.

Studying symptomatic naturally infected dogs without history or clinical evidence of colitis, Adamama-Moraitou et al. (2007) detected, by colonoscopy, patches of hyperemic, edematous, irregular, and mildly erosive colonic mucosa in 25.8% of 31 the animals. Biopsies were obtained and *Leishmania* amastigotes were detected by immunohistochemistry in 32.3% of the dogs. The most common inflammatory pattern in the colonic mucosa of these dogs was pyogranulomatous (90%), whereas dogs without amastigotes did not have any gross or microscopic lesions.

Pinto et al. (2011) performed a systematic study in naturally infected dogs evaluating lesions and parasitological loads in different segments of the gastrointestinal tract, including the stomach, duodenum, jejunum, ileum, cecum and colon. Infected dogs had an increased number of mononuclear cells, but lesions were generally mild. Parasite distribution was evident in all intestinal segments and layers of the gut wall irrespective of the clinical status of the dogs, in accordance to other authors (Toplu & Aydogan, 2011). Interesting, the parasite load was statistically higher in the cecum and colon than in other segments (Pinto et al., 2011), what may explain the most frequently detected diarrhea due to colitis.

Dantas-Torres (2006) reported an intriguing case with the unusual sign of ascites in a dog with symptomatic leishmaniasis in which several free and intracellular amastigotes were found in the peritoneal fluid.

Musculo Skeletical Signs and Lesions

Leishmaniasis has been shown to atypically affect bones, joints and musculature, causing, among others, pain, lameness, stiffness and joints enlargement. Agut et al. (2003) detected orthopedic problems in 44.8% of 26 dogs naturally infected with *L. infantum*. The authors observed that periosteal and intramedullary proliferation were the most common radiographic changes in long bones. In the joints, non-erosive or erosive polyarthritis with soft-tissue swelling were observed. The changes observed in the synovial fluid were associated in most cases with osteolytic lesions. However, *Leishmania* were identified in the synovial fluid from joints without bone radiographic changes (Figure 4).

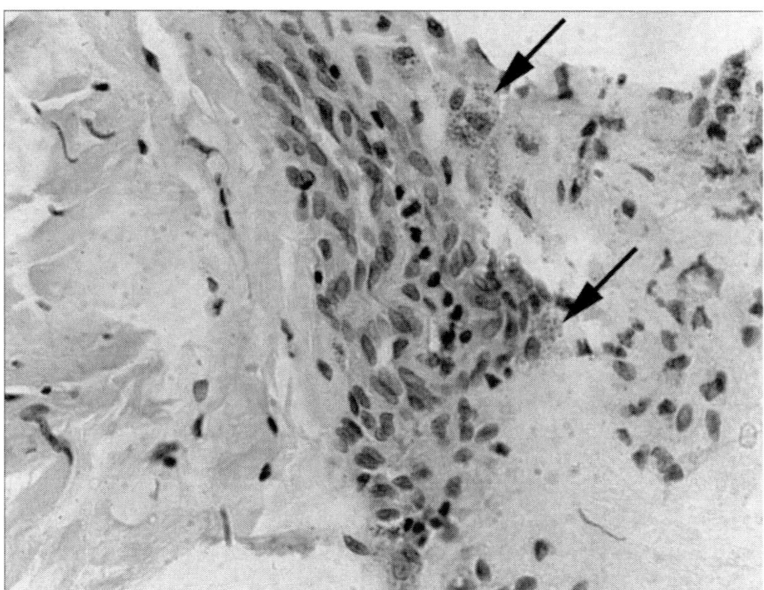

Figure 4. Synovitis in a dog with visceral leishmaniasis. 12-year-old Pinscher bitch with intense focal lympho-histio-plasmacytic inflammatory infiltrate with numerous intracytoplasmic amastigotes within macrophages (arrows). The dog presented osteolysis of the affected joint, confirmed by X-ray and histopathology. HE, 600x.

An interesting case of osteolytic osteomyelitis associated with visceral leishmaniasis was reported by Souza et al. (2005). A dog with a history of weight loss, lymphadenopathy and lameness of the left hind limb was diagnosed with leishmaniasis. Radiological changes of the limb included osteolysis and a periosteal proliferative reaction in the left femoral greater trochanter. These changes were histologically characterized as an osteolytic granulomatous osteomyelitis associated with amastigotes of *Leishmania* within macrophages that were confirmed by immunohistochemistry (Figure 5) and PCR. Another case of intense osteolytic osteomyelitis of the talus and a periosteal reaction of the calcaneus with intralesional amastigotes that required an arthrodesis was reported in a Boxer (Franch et al., 2004).

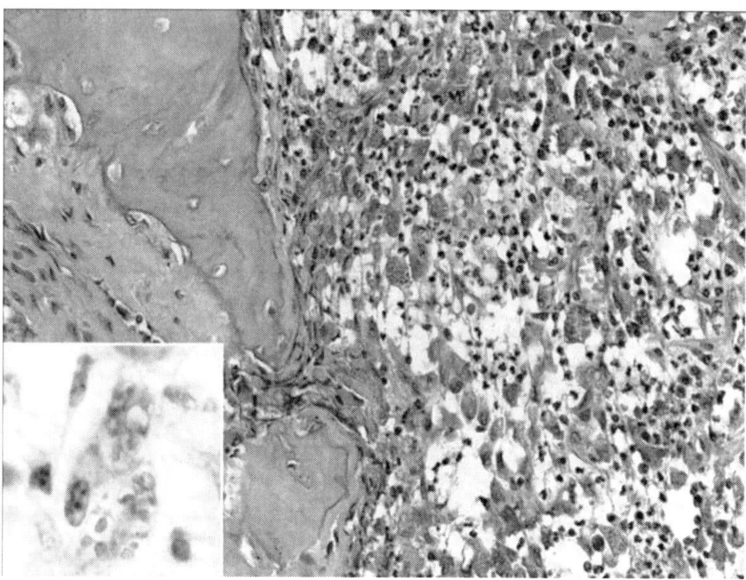

Figure 5. Osteocytic osteomyelitis in a dog with visceral leishmaniasis. 6-month-old male Boxer with intense diffuse granulomatous inflammatory infiltrate with numerous intramacrophagic amastigotes. HE, 400x. In detail, numerous intracytoplasmic positive immunostained amastigotes. IHC – Streptavidin-peroxidase complex, 1000x.

Non immune-mediated polyarthritis, associated or not with systemic leishmaniasis, has also been described, always with the presence of amastigotes in the synovial liquid. Dogs presented stiffness, swollen, and pain during palpation of the joints (Spreng, 1993, Buracco et al., 1997, McConkey et al., 2002).

Paciello et al. (2009) conducted a comprehensive study of muscle biopsies from infected dogs. Mononuclear cells were present with an endomysial, perimysial and perivascular distribution. Various stages of myonecrosis and phagocytosis were observed and invasion of non-necrotic muscle fibers by inflammatory cells was also observed. Atrophic, hypertrophic fibers and muscle regeneration were also found.

The authors showed that *Leishmania* is present within macrophages and not muscle fibers, but can cause myositis due to immunological alterations. Interestingly, there was a direct correlation between the severity of pathological changes, clinical signs and the number of *Leishmania* amastigotes. Earlier, Vamvakidis et al. (2000) had already shown muscle fiber necrosis and atrophy, mononuclear infiltrates and neutrophilic vasculitis in muscles associated with leishmaniasis. Furthermore, IgG immune complexes were detected in muscle samples.

Genital Signs and Lesions

A comprehensive study of genital lesions of infected male dogs demonstrated a very high frequency of inflammatory lesions with intralesional amastigotes particularly in the epididymis (Figure 6), glans penis and prepuce, especially of symptomatic dogs (Diniz et al., 2005). Furthermore, infected dogs shed *Leishmania* in the semen (Riera & Valladares, 1996, Diniz et al., 2005).

A similar study in bitches that analyzed vulva, vagina, cervix, uterine body, uterine horns, uterine tubes and ovaries, demonstrated that vulvar dermatitis was the only important finding in the female genital system, suggesting that *Leishmania* does not have a tropism for these latter tissues (Silva et al., 2008). Importantly, venereal transmission of *Leishmania* from infected dogs to uninfected bitches has been experimentally demonstrated (Silva et al., 2009).

Dubey et al. (2005) reported a case of abortion caused by necrotizing placentitis with numerous intralesional *Leishmania* . However, a later study with eight pregnant bitches did not detect any gross or microscopic findings in the placenta, but amastigotes were detected by immunohistochemistry and PCR in placenta and lymphoreticular tissues from fetus (Pangrazio et al., 2009).

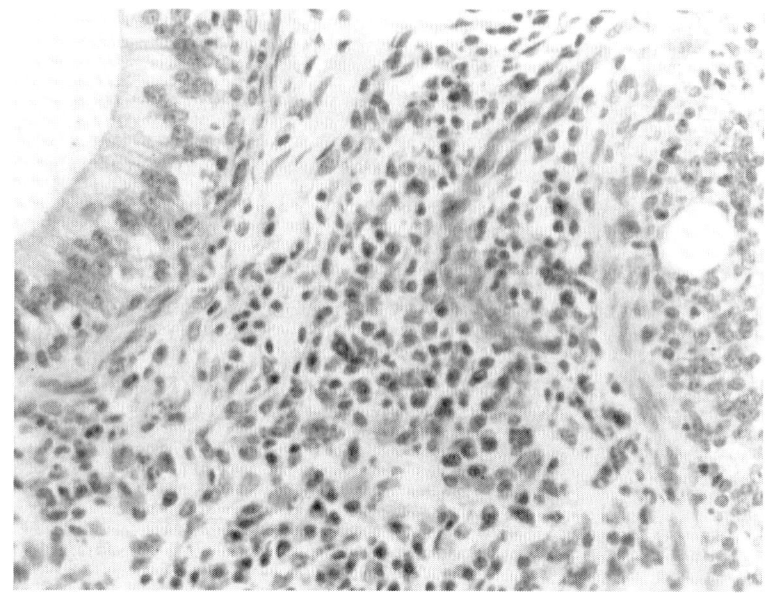

Figure 6. Epididymitis in a dog with visceral leishmaniasis. Adult male mongrel dog with mild diffuse lympho-histio-plasmacytic infiltrate, withintracytoplasmic positive immunostained amastigotes. IHC – Streptavidin-peroxidase complex, 400x.

NERVOUS SIGNS AND LESIONS

Dogs with leishmaniasis may present neurological signs that, according to some authors, may have vascular causes. Nieto et al. (1996) reported an interesting case of leishmaniasis with non-suppurative choroiditis with amastigotes in the choroid plexus. The dog presented lethargy and extreme weakness. Pumarola et al. (1991) described obliterating thrombosis in the lumen of vessels in the choroid plexus of one infected dog, whereas Melo & Machado (2009) reported a significant inflammatory cell infiltration in the brain of dogs infected by *L. infantum*, primarily located in the choroid plexus, subventricular zone and around parenchymal blood vessels. Additionally, multiple foci of vasculitis in spinal cord blood vessels have been shown to cause ischemia, with associated hemorrhage, and subsequent paraplegia in a dog (Font et al., 2004). José-López et al. (2012) reported two cases of leishmaniotic dogs with clinical signs and magnetic resonance imaging findings compatible with multiple brain infarcts. As leishmaniasis can clearly cause cerebrovascular alterations, such as vasculitis, the authors rose the possibility of leishmaniasis predisposing to brain infarcts and other neurological manifestations.

Investigating the nervous system of infected dogs, Garcia-Alonso et al. (1996b) revealed that the cerebrospinal fluid contained anti-*Leishmania* IgG. Also, the encephalon and cerebellum of these dogs presented a pathological sponge-like reaction accompanied by neuronal degeneration, mobilization of glial cells together with accumulation of amyloid deposits. The authors suggested that the interstitial and intravascular deposition of IgG and *Leishmania* antigens in choroid plexus can cause a failure of the blood-cerebrospinal and ciliary bodies filtration barriers. Inflammatory mononuclear infiltrate in brain has been associated with high titers of anti-*Leishmania* antibodies in the cerebrospinal fluid (Melo et al., 2009). In addition, T lymphocyte infiltration has been correlated with cerebrospinal fluid anti-*Leishmania* antibody titres and increase of density of microglia in the ependymal/subependymal area (Melo & Machado, 2011). The authors suggested a pro-inflammatory state in the brains of infected dogs, in which microglia and astrocytes are involved in the pathogenesis of the neurological disorders of visceral leishmaniasis. However, no amastigote was detected in neither of the studies.

There is also a report of *L. infantum* causing meningitis in two dogs (Viñuelas et al., 2001). Granulomatous meningitis was observed with important lympho-plasmacytic inflammatory infiltrate and numerous parasites inside and outside macrophages.

CUTANEOUS LESIONS

Though cutaneous lesions are often present in canine visceral leishmaniasis, unusual manifestations include nodular disease, sterile pustular dermatitis, discoloration of the external nares without ulceration and nodular dermatofibrosis (Ferrer et al., 1988, Koutinas et al., 1992, Ciaramella et al., 1997).

Cavalcanti et al. (2012) reported a curious case in which there were only cutaneous lesions, such as erosive lesions in the limbs, nasal ulcers and seborrheic dermatitis, without systemic manifestations of *L. infantum* infection. Cytology in this case demonstrated a pyogranulomatous inflammation, which was histologically characterized by a necrotizing dermatitis with intralesional amastigotes. This case indicates the importance of not excluding *L. infantum* infection in primary cutaneous manifestations.

Other Manifestations

Unusually, leishmaniasis can be associated to endocrine disorders. A case of primary hypothyroidism clinical and laboratory confirmed was associated with leishmaniasis. Thyroid biopsy showed many *Leishmania* amastigotes, both inside and outside macrophages, causing follicular atrophy and, therefore, low production of thyroid hormones (Cortese et al., 1999).

Interestingly, *Leishmania* amastigotes have been observed within canine transmissible venereal tumor in infected dogs (Albanese et al., 2002, Catone et al., 2003). Therefore, the clinicopathological significance of this association was investigated (Marino et al., 2012). The tumor tends to manifest with a large size and often aggressive behavior in dogs with leishmaniasis. Furthermore, no predictive sign of spontaneous regression was observed, which differs from what is usually observed in non leishmaniotic dogs.

Conclusion

Although canine visceral leishmaniasis has a classical manifestation, atypical signs can be found, making diagnosis a real challenge. The list of manifestations described here may become outdated due to the multifaceted characteristic of the disease. It is very important for clinicians to include leishmaniasis in the differential diagnosis of atypical manifestations, especially in regions where the disease is endemic.

References

Adamama-Moraitou KK, Rallis TS, Koytinas AF, Tontis D, Plevraki K, Kritsepi M. Asymptomatic colitis in naturally infected dogs with *Leishmania infantum*: a prospective study. *Am J Trop Med Hyg*. 2007 Jan;76(1):53-7.

Agut A, Corzo N, Murciano J, Laredo FG, Soler M. Clinical and radiographic study of bone and joint lesions in 26 dogs with leishmaniasis. *Vet Rec*. 2003 Nov;153(21):648-52.

Albanese F, Poli A, Millanta F, Abramo F. Primary cutaneous extragenital canine transmissible venereal tumour with *Leishmania*-laden neoplastic cells: a further suggestion of histiocytic origin? *Vet Dermatol.* 2002 Oct;13(5):243-6.

Alves GB, Pinho FA, Silva SM, Cruz MS, Costa FA. Cardiac and pulmonary alterations in symptomatic and asymptomatic dogs infected naturally with *Leishmania (Leishmania) chagasi. Braz J Med Biol Res.* 2010 Mar;43(3):310-5.

Baneth G, Koutinas AF, Solano-Gallego L, Bourdeau P, Ferrer L. Canine leishmaniosis - new concepts and insights on an expanding zoonosis: part one. *Trends Parasitol.* 2008 Jul;24(7):324-30.

Blavier A, Keroack S, Denerolle P, Goy-Thollot I, Chabanne L, Cadoré JL, et al. Atypical forms of canine leishmaniosis. *Vet J.* 2001 Sep;162(2):108-20.

Bourdoiseau G. Ulcerative glossitis in a dog with leishmaniasis. *Vet Rec.* 2002 Sep;151(11):336.

Buracco P, Abate O, Guglielmino R, Morello E. Osteomyelitis and arthrosynovitis associated with *Leishmania donovani* infection in a dog. *J Small Anim Pract.* 1997 Jan;38(1):29-30.

Carvalho Neta AV, Paixão TA, Silva FL, Santos RL. Panophthalmitis in a dog with visceral leishmaniasis: a case report. *Clínica Veterinária.* 2007 Feb;66.

Catone G, Marino G, Poglayen G, Gramiccia M, Ludovisi A, Zanghì A. Canine transmissible venereal tumour parasitized by *Leishmania infantum. Vet Res Commun.* 2003 Oct;27(7):549-53.

Cavalcanti A, Lobo R, Cupolillo E, Bustamante F, Porrozzi R. Canine cutaneous leishmaniasis caused by neotropical *Leishmania infantum* despite of systemic disease: A case report. *Parasitol Int.* 2012 May.

Ciaramella P, Oliva G, Luna RD, Gradoni L, Ambrosio R, Cortese L, et al. A retrospective clinical study of canine leishmaniasis in 150 dogs naturally infected by *Leishmania infantum. Vet Rec.* 1997 Nov;141(21):539-43.

Cortese L, Oliva G, Ciaramella P, Persechino A, Restucci B. Primary hypothyroidism associated with leishmaniasis in a dog. *J Am Anim Hosp Assoc.* 1999 Nov-Dec;35(6):487-92.

Dantas-Torres F. Presence of *Leishmania* amastigotes in peritoneal fluid of a dog with leishmaniasis from Alagoas, Northeast *Brazil. Rev Inst Med Trop Sao Paulo.* 2006 Jul-Aug;48(4):219-21.

Diniz SA, Melo MS, Borges AM, Bueno R, Reis BP, Tafuri WL, et al. Genital lesions associated with visceral leishmaniasis and shedding of *Leishmania* sp. in the semen of naturally infected dogs. *Vet Pathol.* 2005 Sep;42(5):650-8.

Dubey JP, Rosypal AC, Pierce V, Scheinberg SN, Lindsay DS. Placentitis associated with leishmaniasis in a dog. *J Am Vet Med Assoc.* 2005 Oct;227(8):1266-9, 50.

Ferrer L, Juanola B, Ramos JA, Ramis A. Chronic colitis due to *Leishmania* infection in two dogs. *Vet Pathol.* 1991 Jul;28(4):342-3.

Ferrer L, Rabanal R, Fondevila D, Ramos JA, Domingo M. Skin lesions in canine leishmaniasis. *J Small Anim Pract.* 1988:29:381–8.

Foglia Manzillo V, Pagano A, Paciello O, Di Muccio T, Gradoni L, Oliva G. Papular-like glossitis in a dog with leishmaniosis. *Vet Rec.* 2005 Feb;156(7):213-5.

Foglia Manzillo V, Paparcone R, Cappiello S, De Santo R, Bianciardi P, Oliva G. Resolution of tongue lesions caused by *Leishmania infantum* in a dog treated with the association miltefosine-allopurinol. *Parasit Vectors.* 2009;2 Suppl 1:S6.

Font A, Mascort J, Altimira J, Closa JM, Vilafranca M. Acute paraplegia associated with vasculitis in a dog with leishmaniasis. *J Small Anim Pract.* 2004 Apr;45(4):199-201.

Franch J, Pastor J, Torrent E, Lafuente P, Diaz-Bertrana MC, Munilla A, et al. Management of leishmanial osteolytic lesions in a hypothyroid dog by partial tarsal arthrodesis. *Vet Rec.* 2004 Oct;155(18):559-62.

García-Alonso M, Blanco A, Reina D, Serrano FJ, Alonso C, Nieto CG. Immunopathology of the uveitis in canine leishmaniasis. *Parasite Immunol.* 1996a Dec;18(12):617-23.

Garcia-Alonso M, Nieto CG, Blanco A, Requena JM, Alonso C, Navarrete I. Presence of antibodies in the aqueous humour and cerebrospinal fluid during *Leishmania* infections in dogs. Pathological features at the central nervous system. *Parasite Immunol.* 1996b Nov;18(11):539-46.

Gonçalves R, Tafuri WL, Melo MN, Raso P. Chronic interstitial pneumonitis in dogs naturally infected with *Leishmania (Leishmania) chagasi*: a histopathological and morphometric study. *Rev Inst Med Trop Sao Paulo.* 2003 May-Jun;45(3):153-8.

José-López R, la Fuente CD, Añor S. Presumed brain infarctions in two dogs with systemic leishmaniasis. *J Small Anim Pract.* 2012 Aug.

Koutinas AF, Scott DW, Kantos V, Lekkas S. Skin lesions in canine leishmaniosis (kala-azar): a clinical and histopathological study on 22 spontaneous cases in Greece. *Vet Derm.* 1992;3:121–30.

Lamothe J, Poujade A. Ulcerative glossitis in a dog with leishmaniasis. *Vet Rec.* 2002 Aug;151(6):182-3.

López-Peña M, Alemañ N, Muñoz F, Fondevila D, Suárez ML, Goicoa A, et al. Visceral leishmaniasis with cardiac involvement in a dog: a case report. *Acta Vet Scand.* 2009;51:20.

Marino G, Gaglio G, Zanghì A. Clinicopathological study of canine transmissible venereal tumour in leishmaniotic dogs. *J Small Anim Pract.* 2012 Jun;53(6):323-7.

McConkey SE, López A, Shaw D, Calder J. Leishmanial polyarthritis in a dog. *Can Vet J.* 2002 Aug;43(8):607-9.

Melo GD, Machado GF. Choroid plexus involvement in dogs with spontaneous visceral leishmaniasis: a histopathological investigation. *Braz J Vet Pathol.* 2009:2(2):69-74.

Melo GD, Machado GF. Glial reactivity in dogs with visceral leishmaniasis: correlation with T lymphocyte infiltration and with cerebrospinal fluid anti-*Leishmania* antibody titres. *Cell Tissue Res.* 2011 Dec;346(3):293-304.

Melo GD, Marcondes M, Vasconcelos RO, Machado GF. Leukocyte entry into the CNS of *Leishmania chagasi* naturally infected dogs. *Vet Parasitol.* 2009 Jun;162(3-4):248-56.

Naranjo C, Fondevila D, Leiva M, Roura X, Peña T. Characterization of lacrimal gland lesions and possible pathogenic mechanisms of keratoconjunctivitis sicca in dogs with leishmaniosis. *Vet Parasitol.* 2005 Oct;133(1):37-47.

Naranjo C, Fondevila D, Leiva M, Roura X, Peña T. Detection of *Leishmania* spp. and associated inflammation in ocular-associated smooth and striated muscles in dogs with patent leishmaniosis. *Vet Ophthalmol.* 2010 May;13(3):139-43.

Nieto CG, Viñuelas J, Blanco A, Garcia-Alonso M, Verdugo SG, Navarrete I. Detection of *Leishmania infantum* amastigotes in canine choroid plexus. *Vet Rec.* 1996 Oct;139(14):346-7.

Paciello O, Oliva G, Gradoni L, Manna L, Manzillo VF, Wojcik S, et al. Canine inflammatory myopathy associated with *Leishmania Infantum* infection. *Neuromuscul Disord.* 2009 Feb;19(2):124-30.

Pangrazio KK, Costa EA, Amarilla SP, Cino AG, Silva TM, Paixão TA, et al. Tissue distribution of *Leishmania chagasi* and lesions in transplacentally infected fetuses from symptomatic and asymptomatic naturally infected bitches. *Vet Parasitol.* 2009 Nov;165(3-4):327-31.

Parpaglia ML, Vercelli A, Cocco R, Zobba R, Manunta ML. Nodular lesions of the tongue in canine leishmaniosis. *J Vet Med A Physiol Pathol Clin Med.* 2007 Oct;54(8):414-7.

Peña MT, Naranjo C, Klauss G, Fondevila D, Leiva M, Roura X, et al. Histopathological features of ocular leishmaniosis in the dog. *J Comp Pathol*. 2008 Jan;138(1):32-9.

Peña MT, Roura X, Davidson MG. Ocular and periocular manifestations of leishmaniasis in dogs: 105 cases (1993-1998). *Vet Ophthalmol*. 2000;3(1):35-41.

Pinto AJ, Figueiredo MM, Silva FL, Martins T, Michalick MS, Tafuri WL. Histopathological and parasitological study of the gastrointestinal tract of dogs naturally infected with *Leishmania infantum*. *Acta Vet Scand*. 2011;53:67.

Pumarola M, Brevik L, Badiola J, Vargas A, Domingo M, Ferrer L. Canine leishmaniasis associated with systemic vasculitis in two dogs. *J Comp Pathol*. 1991 Oct;105(3):279-86.

Riera C, Valladares JE. Viable *Leishmania infantum* in urine and semen in experimentally infected dogs. *Parasitol Today*. 1996 Oct;12(10):412.

Shaw SE, Hillman T, Wray J. Unusual case of canine leishmaniosis in the UK. *Vet Rec*. 2008 Aug;163(9):283.

Silva FL, Rodrigues AA, Rego IO, Santos RL, Oliveira RG, Silva TM, et al. Genital lesions and distribution of amastigotes in bitches naturally infected with *Leishmania chagasi*. *Vet Parasitol*. 2008 Jan;151(1):86-90.

Silva FL, Oliveira RG, Silva TMA, Xavier MN, Nascimento EF, Santos RL. Venereal transmission of canine visceral leishmaniasis. *Vet Parasitol*. 2009;160:55-9.

Slappendel RJ. Canine leishmaniasis. A review based on 95 cases in The Netherlands. *Vet Q*. 1988 Jan;10(1):1-16.

Souza AI, Juliano RS, Gomes TS, de Araujo Diniz S, Borges AM, Tafuri WL, et al. Osteolytic osteomyelitis associated with visceral leishmaniasis in a dog. *Vet Parasitol*. 2005 Apr;129(1-2):51-4.

Spreng D. Leishmanial polyarthritis in two dogs. *J Small Anim Pract*. 1993;34:559-63.

Toplu N, Aydogan A. An immunohistochemical study in cases with usual and unusual clinicopathological findings of canine visceral leishmaniosis. *Parasitol Res*. 2011 Oct;109(4):1051-7.

Torrent E, Leiva M, Segalés J, Franch J, Peña T, Cabrera B, et al. Myocarditis and generalised vasculitis associated with leishmaniosis in a dog. *J Small Anim Pract*. 2005 Nov;46(11):549-52.

Vamvakidis CD, Koutinas AF, Kanakoudis G, Georgiadis G, Saridomichelakis M. Masticatory and skeletal muscle myositis in canine leishmaniasis (*Leishmania infantum*). *Vet Rec*. 2000 Jun;146(24):698-703.

Viegas C, Requicha J, Albuquerque C, Sargo T, Machado J, Dias I, et al. Tongue nodules in canine leishmaniosis - a case report. *Parasit Vectors*. 2012;5:120.

Viñuelas J, García-Alonso M, Ferrando L, Navarrete I, Molano I, Mirón C, et al. Meningeal leishmaniosis induced by *Leishmania infantum* in naturally infected dogs. *Vet Parasitol*. 2001 Oct;101(1):23-7.

In: Leishmaniasis
Editor: Carlos Sepulveda

ISBN: 978-1-62417-700-2

Chapter 5

PARASITOLOGICAL, SEROLOGICAL DIAGNOSIS OF CANINEVISCERAL LEISHMANIASIS, ASSOCIATION OF NEUTROPHILIC INFLAMMATORY INFILTRATE AND TRANSMISSION POTENTIAL: A REVIEW

Francisco A. L. Costa,[1*] Aline A. Carvalho,[1] José A. L. Lindoso[2,3†] and Hiro Goto[2,4‡]

[1]Departamento de Clinica e Cirurgia Veterinária, Centro de Ciências Agrárias, Universidade Federal do Piauí,Teresina, Piauí, Brasil

[2]Laboratório de Soroepidemiologia-Instituto de MedicinaTropical de São Paulo, Universidade de São Paulo, SP, Brasil

[*]Corresponding author: Francisco A. L. Costa. Universidade Federal do Piauí. Centro de Ciências Agrárias. Departamento de Clinica e Cirurgia Veterinária. Setor de patologia Animal, 64049-550, Campus Socopo- S/N, Teresina, Piauí, Brasil. Telefone: + 55 86 3215 5760, número do Fax: + 55 86 3215 5753, E-mail: fassisle@gmail.com.

[†]José A. L. Lindoso: Laboratório de Soroepidemiologia-Institutode Medicina Tropical de SãoPaulo. Av. Dr. Enéas de Carvalho, Aguiar 470, prédio II, 4° andar, 05403-000, SP. Instituto de Infectologia Emilio Ribas-SES-SP, Avenida Dr. Arnaldo, 165, 01246-000-São Paulo-SP.

[‡]Hiro Goto: Laboratório de Soroepidemiologia-Instituto de MedicinaTropical de São Paulo, Universidade de São Paulo. Av. Dr. Enéas de Carvalho, Aguiar 470, prédio II, 4° andar, 05403-000, SP, Brasil.

[3]Instituto de Infectologia Emilio Ribas-SES-SP, São Paulo-SP, Brasil
[4]Departamento de Medicina Preventiva, Faculdade de Medicina, Universidade de São Paulo, SP, Brasil

Abstract

Canine visceral leishmaniasis (CVL) is important in the transmission cycle of *Leishmania (Leishmania) infantum* as it constitutes the main reservoir of the parasite in the peridomestic cycle. We revise the laboratory diagnosis of CVL since control program in some parts of the world including Brazil has in its guideline the culling of infected dogs based on anti-*Leishmania* antibody detection. But the serological techniques have limitation regarding the specificity and sensitivity. The confirmation of infection is performed by parasitological analysis that is considered the gold standard since it presents 100% specificity. Whereas sensitivity, specificity and predictive values of the parasitological methods are critical aspects for the diagnosis of CVL per se and for the dogs as source of parasite for transmission, parameters that may give indication of this potential are important to unveil. Here we discuss the serological diagnosis and then the parasitological diagnosis with focus on neutrophilic infiltrate in the tissue related to transmission potential.

Keywords: Lymph nodes, skin, neutrophil, parasite load, *Leishmania*

Introduction

Visceral leishmaniasis (VL) is caused in Brazil by *Leishmania (Leishmania) infantum* (Mauricio et al., 2001). The diagnosis of canine VL (CVL) is difficult beginning from the clinical approach given that the dogs present symptoms similar to babesiosis, hepatozoonosis, heartworm, ancilostomoses (Kontos; Koutinas, 1993) and ehrlichiosis (Font et al., 1993). Here we discuss the laboratory approaches for the diagnosis of CVL with their impediments.

From the epidemiological stand point CVL is important due to its high prevalence and greater potential for spreading the disease as it constitutes the main reservoir of *Leishmania (Leishmania) infantum*in the peridomestic cycle. Infected dogs have parasites in the skin that are potentially transmissible for the vector (Traviet al., 2001; Moreno; Alvar, 2002; Reis et al., 2009).

The diagnosis of CVL is crucial since VL control program in some parts of the world including Brazil has in its guideline the culling of infected dogs based on anti-*Leishmania* antibody detection. However serological diagnosis presents some pitfalls but still useful in the diagnosis of CVL as we discuss bellow. Since serological assay is indirect method more direct proof of infection is desirable and the confirmation of infection is performed by parasitological analysis on sample aspirate of skin, lymph node and bone marrow (Willense, 1995) for cytological analysis what is considered the gold standard since it presents 100% specificity. Nonetheless the parasitological methods have in general low sensitivity if we consider the entire population of infected dogs due in part to the parasite load that uses to be low when the dogs do not present overt signs of disease (Alvaret al., 2004). Greater sensitivity is achieved when performed on samples obtained by aspiration of lymph node and bone marrow with 30-50% (Ferrer, 1999) and 60-75% (Alvar etal., 2004) positivity, respectively. Alternative to the cytological exam, histopathological analysis of tissue sections stained with hematoxylin-eosin (HE) has also been used to detect amastigotes of the parasite despite its low sensitivity (Xavier et al., 2006). As with cytological technique, the sensitivity is higher when examined by a well experienced professional (Maia; Campino, 2008).

Considering the high specificity of the parasitological technique we may consider its application in endemic area as complementary to serological diagnosis or supporting method for the diagnosis contributing to the reliable and rapid identification of infected animals. Here we discuss the serological diagnosis and then the parasitological diagnosis with focus on neutrophilic infiltrate in the tissue related to transmission potential.

Serological Diagnosis of CVL

Different serological techniques are used in the diagnosis of leishmaniasis: indirect immunofluorescence antibody test (IFAT), direct agglutination test (DAT), Enzyme linked immunosorbent assay (ELISA), Western Blotting (WB) and more recently immunochromatographic test 'disptick'. Except the latter, the techniques employ total antigen, intact parasites or their soluble extracts. Assays with these antigens have limitation regarding the specificity (Badaró et al., 1986; Celeste et al., 1988; Choudhary et al., 1992; Sundar et al., 2002). The assays with high sensitivity as ELISA have problems of specificity with frequent occurrence of false-positive results due to cross-reactivity with other pathogens such as *Babesia canis* (Manciantiet al., 1996), *Trypanosoma congolensis* and *T. evansi* (el Harith, 1989; Vercammen, 1997) and even cross-reactions with *Ehlichia canis* although controversial (Wood and Hoskiins, 1991; Mancianti, 1996; Guillénllera, 2002). The techniques that use intact parasites such as IFAT provide more reproducible and more specific results and therefore the IFAT is considered confirmatory assay for CVL. This assay however depends some way on the technician's subjective evaluation as well as on the parasite culture to prepare the slides for the reaction. In serological surveys it is performed the ELISA with total *Leishmania* antigen for screening with subsequent confirmation of the positive cases with IFAT. Lately recombinant antigens as the K39 (rK39) have been used in immunoenzymatic and rapid immunochromatographic tests (dipsticks) in serological diagnosis of human VL for field or laboratory use (Sundaret al., 1998). These assays in human VL have sensitivity that varies according to the geographic region but high specificity (Cunningham et al., 2012). However the rK39 is a marker of active disease and an evaluation in Brazil on CVL showed high specificity (96%) but low sensitivity (47%) with negative results in many parasitologically positive asymptomatic cases (Grimaldiet al., 2012) what would be a serious problem in the control of CVL since some *Leishmania* transmission control program recommends euthanasia of seropositive dogs even if asymptomatic. Other rapid tests has also been evaluated in the diagnosis of CVL with varied results: the rapid ELISA with 94.7% sensitivity and 90.6% specificity (Marcondeset al., 2011); and the fast agglutination screening test (FAST) and direct agglutination test (DAT) with 98.60% sensitivity and 78.70% specificity (Babakhan et al., 2009).

Serological assays for the diagnosis of CVL has to be improved using recombinant antigens and more sensitive assays developed maybe incorporating new markers to enable the detection of asymptomatic dogs.

Parasitological Diagnosis of CVL and Its Relationship to Neutrophilic Inflammatory Infiltrate

Whereas sensitivity, specificity and predictive values of the parasitological methods are critical aspects for the diagnosis of CVL per se and for the dogs as source of parasite for transmission, parameters that may give indication of this potential are important to unveil. It is still a matter of controversy whether asymptomatic dogs are important source for transmission of *L. (L.) infantum* to humans thus we have been analyzing symptoms, parasite load and transmission potential in VL dogs from endemic area to contribute to this discussion. In this issue, in asymptomatic dogs infected by *Leishmania (L.) infantum* it has been shown low parasitism in organs from mononuclear phagocytic system and even absence of parasites in the skin (Solano-Gallego et al., 2001) what we also confirmed in a previous study. Asymptomatic dog presented low parasitism in the skin with negative xenodiagnosis showing low or no transmission potential (Table 1) with opposite finding in symptomatic dogs (Verçosa et al., 2008).

Table 1. Clinical signs, xenodiagonosis and inflammatory infiltrate in 23 *Leishmania (L.) infantum*-naturally infected serologically and parasitologically positive dogs

Animals	Skin lesions	Adenopathy	Xenodiagnosis	Inflammatory infiltrate		
				Lymphocyte/ Macrophage	Plasma cells	PMN
S1	+	+	+	+++	+++	-
S2	+	+	+	+++	+++	+
S3	+	+	-	+++	+++	+
S4	+	-	-	+++	-	+++
S5	+	+	+	+++	+	+++
S6	+	+	+	+++	-	+++
S7	-	+	nd	+++	-	+++
S8	-	-	-	+++	+++	+
S9	+	+	+	+++	+++	+
S10	+	+	+	+++	-	+
S11	+	-	nd	+++	-	-
S12	+	-	nd	+++	-	-
As1	-	-	nd	+++	+++	-
As2	-	-	-	+++	+++	-
As3	-	-	-	+++	-	-
As4	-	-	-	+++	-	-
As5	-	-	-	+++	-	-
As6	-	-	nd	+++	-	-
As7	-	-	nd	+++	-	-
As8	-	-	nd	+++	-	-
As9	-	-	nd	+++	-	-
As10	-	-	nd	+++	-	-
As11	-	-	-	-	-	-

S1 – S12 = symptomatic dog; As1 – As11 = asymptomatic dog; nd = not done. PMN = polymorphonuclear neutrophils. Adapted from Verçosa et al., 2008.

Table 2. Detection of amastigote in the *imprint* of lymph nodes and in skin biopsy of polysymptomatic and oligosymptomatic dogs naturally infected by *Leishmania (Leishmania) infantum*

Cytological Exam	Polysymptomatic	Oligosymptomatic	Total
Lymph node imprint	26 (81.2%)	15 (48.3%)	41 (65.1%)
Skin biopsy	17 (53.1%)	05 (16.1%)	22 (34.9%)
Total			63 (100.0%)

One aspect that we considered interesting in the histopathological exam of the skin in this study was the prominent presence of polymorphonuclear neutrophils (PMN) in the inflammatory infiltrate in those dogs that had positive xenodiagnosis (Table 1). Based on these results we have studied the possible improvement of parasitological diagnosis combining search for parasites and histopathological parameters with focus on neutrophil infiltrate in easily accessible samples in dogs. The PMN infiltrate may constitute a potential indicator of the presence of the parasite contributing to the search of *Leishmania* in tissue samples and their concomitant presence may indicate a transmission potential of these animals.

Recently we analized the skin and popliteal lymph node of polysymptomatic and oligosymptomatic dogs. The parasitological analysis in all seropositive dogs showed amastigotes in the lymph nodes in 65.1% (41/63) and in the skin in 39.7% (25/63) (Table 2) and these were all positive in lymph node. In other studies higher frequency of positivity was in the skin (Pinho, 2010) that may be explained by the clinical conditions of the animals more severily ill since it is well known that animals that have more parasites in the skin are usually polysymptomatic (Queirozet al.,2010).

In a set of infected dogs (N = 20) parasite load was evaluated and we observed significantly higher load in polysymptomatic than in oligo-symptomatic dogs on both the skin ($p < 0.05$, KruskalWallis and Newman Keuls Student) and the lymph node ($p < 0.05$, Kruskal Wallis and Dunn's method). In these animals the clinical findings were lymphadenopathy (70%), onychogryphosis (70%), conjunctivitis (50%), skin peeling (30%), alopecia (30%), weight loss (30%), ulceration skin (20%), pale mucous membranes (20%), limb edema (15%), depigmentation of the nose (10%) and epistaxis (5%) and there was a direct correlation between the parasite load in the lymph node and the number of clinical signs ($p < 0.05$, $r = 0.7$, linear regression) (Figure 1).

This probably reflects the state of disease progression and increased risk of infection transmission. Similarly this relationship was observed in another study between parasitism and severity of skin manifestations (Queirozet al., 2011) while some others have shown no correlation (Lima et al., 2004; Giunchettiet al., 2008).

In ear skin and popliteal lymph node of these animals cytological exam was performed to quantify the presence of neutrophils. We observed a positive correlation between the parasite load and the amount of neutrophils ($p < 0.05$, $r = 0.7$, regression analysis) in ear skin (Figure 2A) as well as in the popliteal lymph node of infected dogs ($p< 0.05$, $r = 0.6$, Linear Regression) (Figure2B).

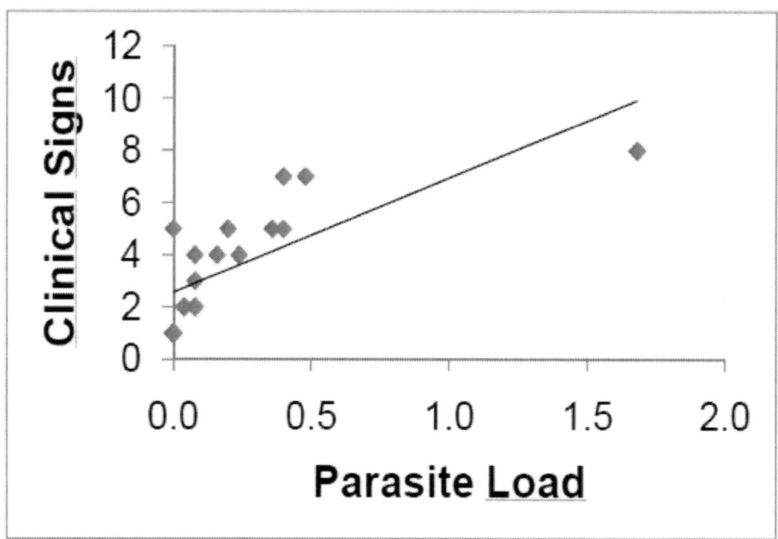

Figure 1.Correlation between the parasite load in lymph nodes and the number of clinical signs of dogs naturally infected by *Leishmania (Leishmania) infantum*.$p< 0.05$, Linear Regression.

In histopathological analysis of the ear skin of 10 polysymptomatic dogs we observed subepidermal and periannexal diffuse and focal inflammatory infiltrate constituted by mononuclear cells (macrophages and lymphocytes) but also neutrophils (Figure 3A). In the infiltrate eosinophils, plasma cells and fibroblasts were also seen. In three dogs severe inflammatory infiltrate extending to the dermis with focal granulomatous accumulation of mononuclear cells (Figure3B) was seen.

In oligosymptomatic dogs subepidermal and periannexal inflammatory infiltrate was also observed constituted by mononuclear cells (macrophages, lymphocytes) but rare eosinophils (Figure 3C).

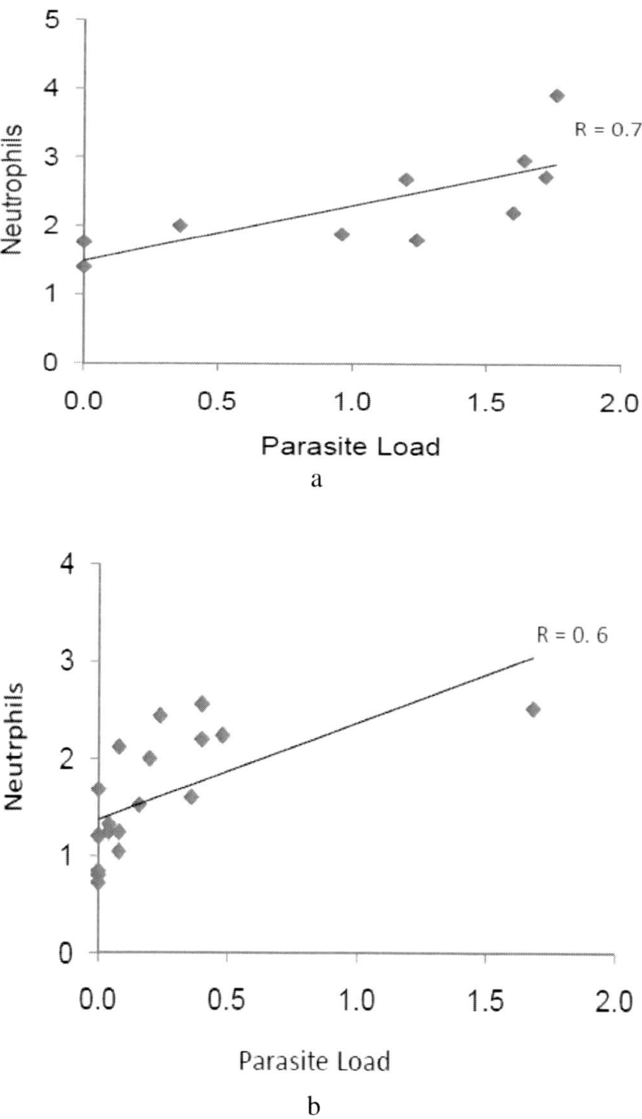

Figure 2. Correlation between parasite load and neutrophils in skin of ear (A) and popliteal lymph nodes (B) of dogs naturally infected by *Leishmania (Leishmania) infantum*. $p < 0.05$, Linear Regression.

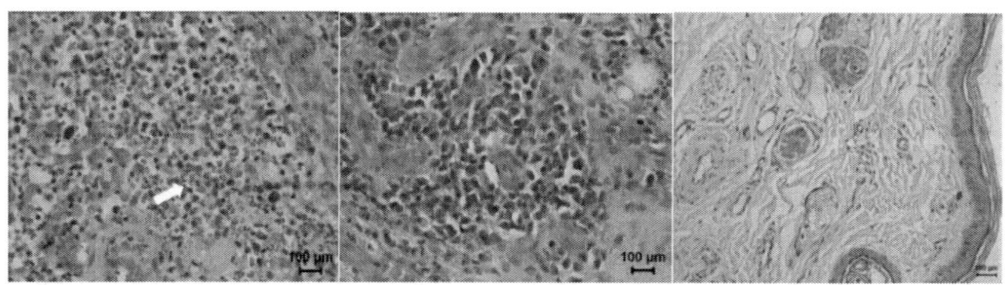

Figure 3. Histological section of the skin of ear of dog naturally infected by *Leishmania (Leishmania) infantum*. (A) Inflammatory infiltrate with presence of neutrophils (arrows). (B) Granuloma. (C) Mononuclear inflammatory infiltrate without neutrophils. H-E staining. Magnification: 40x.

The role of neutrophils during *Leishmania* infection is controversial. Neutrophils are the first cells that migrate to the site of infection and actively phagocytize and kill the parasites (Pearson and Steigbiegel, 1981). In this line, the importance of neutrophils in the initial control of *Leishmania* major infection was determined in neutrophil-deficient mice which showed exacerbation of the lesion of the foot pad (Lima et al., 1998).

Conversely in another study the parasites were shown viable within neutrophils (Peters et al., 2008) suggesting their involvement in the progressionof infection functioning as 'Trojan horse' when internalized by macrophages where the parasites would proliferate (Gueirardet al., 2008).

Seemingly neutrophil phagocytosis may also occurs without formation of fagolysosome when the parasites are not destroyed involving phosphoglican in the suppression of apoptosis of infected neutrophils prolonging their longevity in the cells (Aga et al. 2002).

It has also been shown that necrotic or apoptotic neutrophils contribute to the proliferation of *Leishmania* within macrophages in susceptible mouse strains (Ribeiro-Gomes et al., 2004). Another interesting finding is that in susceptible mouse strains the neutrophil infiltrate in the skin lesion lasts longer than in resistant mouse strains (Beilet al., 1992) an aspect that deserves further studies.

We have observed a positive correlation between parasite load and the presence of neutrophils in the skin and popliteal lymph node. This correlation was most obvious in polysymptomatic than in oligosymptomatic dogs. These results suggest that the presence of neutrophils contributes to the progression of infection as suggested by studies in mouse models.

Conclusion

For the diagnosis of CVL serological assays may improve with the use of recombinant antigens and of markers to improve the sensitivity. Concerning parasitological diagnosis based on the finding of parasites and the characteristics of the inflammatory infiltrate with or without neutrophils in the analysis of lymph node smear we may infer the potential epidemiological risk of a dog to transmit the parasite to the vector. The presence of few neutrophils in lymph node smear is indication of low parasite burden in the skin. In opposition it is high when greater the neutrophils in the infiltrate.

References

Aga, E.; Katschinski, D. M.; Zandbergen, G.; Laufs, L.; Hansen, L.; Müller, K.; Solbach, W.; Laskay, T. 2002. Inhibition of the spontaneous apoptosis of neutrophil granulocytes by the intracellular parasite *Leishmaniamajor*. *J. Immunol.* v.169, p. 898-905.

Alvar, J.; Canavate, C.; Molina, R.; Moreno, J.; Nieto, J. 2004. Canine leishmaniasis. *Advances in Parasitol.* v.57, p. 1-88.

Babakhan, L.; Mohebali, M.; Akhoundi, B.; Edrissian, G.H.; Keshavarz, H. 2009. Rapid detection of *Leishmania infantum* infection in dogs: a comparative study using fast agglutination screening test (FAST) and direct agglutination test (DAT) in Iran. *Parasitol. Res.* v. 105, p. 717-20.

Badaró, R.; Reed, S.G.; Barral, A.; Orge, G.; Jones, T.C. 1986. Evaluation of the microenzyme linked immunosorbent assay (ELISA) for antibodies in american visceral leishmaniasis: antigen seletion for detection of infection specific responses. *Am. J. Trop. Med. Hyg.* v. 35, p. 72-78.

Beil, W.J.; Meinardus-Hager, G.; Neugebauer, D.C.; Sorg, C. 1992. Differences in the onset of the inflammatory response to cutaneous leishmaniasis in resistant and susceptible mice. *J. Leukoc. Biol.* v. 52, p. 135-42.

Celeste, B.J.; Guimarães, M.C.S.; Corrales, L.E.M. 1988. Peroxidase antibody test for mucocutaneous leishmaniasis serology performance indexes and comparison with a fluorescent antibody test. *Rev. Inst. Med. Trop. São Paulo.* v. 30, p. 411-417.

Choudhary, A.; Puri, A.; Guru, P.Y.; Saxena, K.C. 1992. An indirect fluorescent antibody (IFA) test for the serodiagnosis of kalazar. *J. Commun. Dis.* v. 24, p. 32-36.

Cunningham, J.; Hasker, E.; Das, P.; El Safi, S.; Goto, H.; Mondal, D.; Mbuchi, M.; Mukhtar, M.; Rabello, A.; Rijal, S.; Sundar, S.; Wasunna, M.; Adams, E.; Menten, J.; Peeling, R.; Boelaert, M. for the WHO/TDR Visceral Leishmaniasis Laboratory Network. 2012. A Global Comparative Evaluation of Commercial Immunochromatographic Rapid Diagnostic Tests for Visceral Leishmaniasis. *Clin. Infect. Dis.* v. 55, p. 1312-1319.

El Harith, A.; Slappendel, R.J.; Reiter, I.; van Knapen, F.; de Korte, P.; Huigen, E.; Kolk, A.H. 1989. Application of a direct agglutination test for detection of specific anti-*Leishmania* antibodies in the canine reservoir. *J. Clin. Microbiol.* v. 27, p. 2252-7.

Ferrer, L. M. 1999. Clinical aspect of leishmaniasis In: *Proceedings or the International Canine Leishmaniasis Forum Barcelona, Spain.* Canine Leishmaniasis on update: Wiesbaden Hoeschst Roussel Vet. p. 6-10.

Font, A.; Closa, J. M.; Molina, A.; Mascort, J. 1993. Trombosis and nephotic syndrome in a dog with visceral leishmaniasis. *The Journal of Small Animal Practice.* v. 34, p. 446-470.

Giunchetti, R. C.; Martins-Filho, O. A.; Carneiro, C. M.; Mayrink, W.; Marques, M. J.; Tafuri, W. L.; Corrêia-Oliveira, R.; Reis, A. B. 2008. Histopathology, parasite density and cell phenotypes of the popliteal lymph node in canine visceral leishmaniasis. *Vet. Immunol. Immunopathol.* v.121, p. 23-33.

Grimaldi, G. Jr.; Teva, A.; Ferreira, A. L.; dos Santos, C.B.; Pinto, I.S.; de-Azevedo, C.T.; Falqueto, A. 2012. Evaluation of a novel chromatographic immunoassay based on Dual-Path Platform technology (DPP® CVL rapidtest) for the serodiagnosis of canine visceral leishmaniasis. *Trans. R. Soc. Trop. Med. Hyg.* v. 106, p. 54-9.

Gueirard, P.; Laplante, A.; Rondeau, C.; Milon, G.; Desjardins, M. 2008. Trafficking of *Leishmania donovani* promastigotes in non-lytic compartments in neutrophils enables the subsequent transfer of parasite to macrophages. *Cell. Microbiol.* v.10, p. 100-111.

Guillenllera, J.L.; Lopez Garcia, M.L.; Martin Reinoso, E.; De Vivar Gonzalez, R. 2002. Differential serological testing by simultaneous indirect immunofluorescent antibody test in canine leishmaniosis and ehrlichiosis. *Vet. Parasitol.* v. 109, p. 185-90.

Kontos, V.J.; Koutinas, A.F. 1993. Old world canine leishmaniasis. *Continuing Education Articles*. v. 15, p. 949-959.

Lima, W.G.; Michalick, M.S.M.; Melo, M.N.; Tafuri, W.L.; Tafuri, W.L. 2004. Canine visceral leishmaniasis: a histopathological study of lymph nodes. *Acta Tropica*. v. 92, p. 43-53.

Lima, G. M.; Vallochi, A. L.; Silva, U. R.; Bevilacqua, E. M.; Kiffer, M. M.; Abrahamsohn, I. A. 1998. The role of polymorphonuclear leukocytes in the resistance to cutaneous leishmaniasis. *Immunol. Lett*. v. 64, p. 145–151.

Mancianti, F.; Pedonese, F.; Poli, A. 1996.Evaluation of dot enzyme-linked immunosorbent assay (dot-ELISA) forthe serodiagnosis of canine leishmaniosis as compared with indirect immunofluorescence assay.*Vet. Parasitol*. v. 65, p. 1-9.

Maia, C.; Campino, L. 2008.Methods for diagnosis of canine leishmaniasis and immune response to infection. *Vet. Parasitol*. v. 158, p. 274-287.

Marcondes, M.; Biondo, A.W.; Gomes, A.A.; Silva, A.R.; Vieira, R.F.; Camacho, A.A.; Quinn, J.; Chandrashekar, R. 2011. Validation of a *Leishmaniainfantum* ELISA rapid test for serological diagnosis of *Leishmaniachagasi* in dogs. *Vet. Parasitol*. v. 175, p. 15-9.

Mauricio, I.L.; Gaunt, M.W.; Stothard, J.R.; Miles, M.A. 2001. Genetic typing and phylogeny of the *Leishmania donovani* complex by restriction analysis of PCR amplified gp63 intergenic regions. *Parasitology*. v. 122, p. 393-403.

Moreno, J.; Alvar, J. 2002. Canine leishmaniasis: Epidemiological risk and the experimental model. *Trends Parasitol*. v. 18, p. 399-405.

Pearson, R.D.; Steigbigel, R.T. 1981. Phagocytosis and killing of the protozoan *Leishmania donovani* by human polymorphonuclear leukocytes. *J. Immunol*. v. 127, p. 1438–1443.

Peters, N.C.; Egen, J.G.; Secundino, N.; Debrabant, A.; Kimblin, N.; Kamhawi, S.; Lawyer, P.; Fay, M.P.; Germain, R.N.; Sacks, D. L. 2008. In vivo imaging reveals an essential role for neutrophils in leishmaniasis transmitted by sand flies. *Science*. v. 321, p. 970-974.

Pinho, F. A. Quantificação de mRNA de IGF-I em pele, fígado, baço e linfonodo poplíteo de cães naturalmente infectados por *Leishmania (Leishmania) chagasi,* 2010. Dissertação (Mestrado em ciência animal) - Centro de Ciências Agrárias, Curso de Medicina Veterinária, Universidade Federal do Piauí, Teresina, 2010.

Queiroz, N.M.G.P.; Assis, J.; Oliveira, T.M.F.S.; Machado, R.S.; Nunes, C. M.; Starke-Buzetti, W. A. 2010. Diagnóstico da Leishmaniose Visceral Canina pelas técnicas de imunoistoquímica e PCR em tecidos cutâneos em associação com a RIFI e ELISA-teste. *Rev. Bras. Parasitol. Vet.* v. 1, p. 34-40.

Queiroz, N.M.G.P.; Silveira, R.C.V.; Noronha Jr., A.C.F.; Oliveira, T.M.F.S.; Machado, R.Z.; Starke-Buzetti, W. A. 2011. Detection of *Leishmania (L.) chagasi* in canine skin. *Vet. Parasitol.* v. 178, p. 1-8.

Reis, A.B.; Martins-Filho, O.A.; Teixeira-Carvalho, A.; Giunchetti, R.C.; Carneiro, C.M.; Mayrink, W.;Tafuri, W.L.; Corrêa-Oliveira, R. 2009. Systemic and compartmentalized immune response in canine visceral leishmaniasis.*Vet. Immunol. Immunopathol.* v.128, p. 87-95.

Ribeiro-Gomes, F.L.; Otero, A.C.; Gomes, N.A.; Moniz-De-Souza, M.C.; Cysne-Finkelstein, L.; Arnholdt, A.C.; Calich, V.L.; Coutinho, S.G.; Lopes, M.F.; Dos Reis, G.A. 2004. Macrophage interactions with neutrophils regulate *Leishmania major* infection. *J. Immunol.* v. 172, p. 4454-4462.

Solano-Gallego, L.; Rieira, C.; Roupa, X.; Iniestra, L.; Gallego, M.; Valladares, J. E.; Fisa, R.; Castillejo, S.; Alberola, J.; Ferrer, L. Arboix, M.; Portus, M. 2001. *Leishmania infantum*-specific IgG, IgG1 and IgG2 antibody response in healthy and ill dogs from endemic areas. Evolution in the course of infection and after treatment. *Vet. Parasitol.* v. 96, p. 265-276.

Sundar, S.; Reed, S.G.; Sinh, V.P; Kumar, P.C.; Murray, H.W. 1998. Rapid accurate field diagnosis of Indian visceral leishmaniasis. *Lancet.* v. 351, p. 563-5.

Sundar, S.; Pai, M. 2002. Laboratory diagnosis of visceral leishmaniasis. *Clin. Diag. Lab. Immunol.* v. 9, p. 951-8.

Travi, B.L.; Tabares, C.J.; Cadena, H.; Ferro, C.; Osorio, Y. 2001. Canine visceral leishmaniasis in Colombia: relationship between clinical and parasitologic status and infectivity for sand flies. *Am. J. Trop. Med. Hyg.* v. 64, p. 119-124.

Vercammen, F.; Berkvens, D.; Le Ray, D.; Jacquet, D.; Vervoort, T. 1997. Development of a slide ELISA for canine leishmaniasis and comparison with four serological tests. *Vet. Res.* v. 141, p. 328-30.

Verçosa, B.L.A.; Lemos, C.M.; Mendonça, I.L.; Silva, S.M.M.S.; Carvalho, S.M.; Goto, H.; Costa, F.A.L. 2008. Transmission potencial, skin inflammatory response and parasitism of symptomatic and asymptomatic dogs with visceral leishmaniasis. *BMC Vet. Res.* v. 4, p. 1-7.

Xavier, S.C.; Andrade, H.M.; Hadade Monte, S.J.; Chiarelli, I.M.; Lima, W.G.; Michialick, M.S.; Tafuri, W.L.; Tafuri, W.L. 2006. Comparison of paraffin-embedded skin biopsies from different anatomical regions as sampling methods for detection of *Leishmania* infection in dogs using histological, immunohistochemical and PCR methods. *BMC Vet. Res.* v. 2, p. 1-7.

Woody, B.J.; Hoskins, J.D. 1991. Ehrlichial diseases of dogs. *Vet. Clin. North Am. Small Anim. Pract*. v. 21, p. 75-98.

Willemse, T. Leishmaniose. *Dermatologia Clínica de cães e gatos*. 1ed. São Paulo: Manole, 1995. cap. 5, p. 42-43.

INDEX

A

B

C

D

E

F

G

H

I

J

K

L

M

N

O

S

T

U

V

W